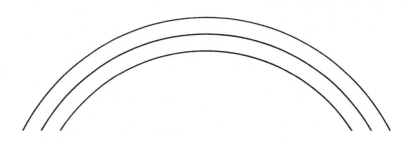

HEALING

THE COMING REVOLUTION

IN HOLISTIC MEDICINE

·

JACK LaPATRA

McGRAW-HILL BOOK COMPANY

New York   St. Louis   San Francisco   Mexico   Toronto   Düsseldorf

Library of Congress Cataloging in Publication Data
LaPatra, Jack W   1927–
Healing: the coming revolution in holistic medicine.
Bibliography: p.
Includes index.
1. Therapeutic systems. 2. Medicine—Philosophy.
3. Mind and body. I. Title. [DNLM: 1. Therapeutic
cults. WB890 L314h]
R733.L36   1978   615.5′01   78-19013
ISBN 0-07-036359-5

1234567890 BPBP 78321098

Published in association with SAN FRANCISCO BOOK COMPANY

To my sister NANCY *with love*

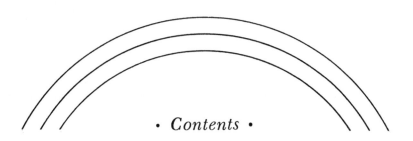

· Contents ·

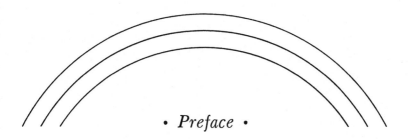

• *Preface* •

Throughout my life I have always been aware of the marvels of modern medicine. As I grew up, news of scientific advances marched into my consciousness, propelled by the media and substantiated by the adults around me. Information about vaccines, drugs, machines, and new operations and treatments came from all directions, and it took me a long time to realize that few of those reports had anything to do with me or anyone I knew. They were like a modern mythology. The main result was that doctors became unreal, god-like figures to me.

I seldom saw physicians, and when I did the meetings were brief and confusing. I was humble in their presence and anxious for a speedy delivery of the prescription that led to the pills which seemed to help. I was raised by my grandparents, who never, in my memory, saw a doctor. In retrospect, I am convinced that they kept me in good health by a combination of wit, wisdom, and intuition. They seemed to know the precise moment when it was appropriate for me to see a doctor. Their wisdom included an array of home remedies gathered from their rural background and a set of basic truths about health. Things like getting plenty of rest and loving attention when I didn't feel well.

I am not a physician, but I have been deeply involved with health professionals for many years. As a professor in a university setting I have studied the delivery of health services for nearly a decade, first in a department of community health, and more recently in a school of health systems. I have written a professional book on the delivery of health services.

Somehow, during the years of these intellectual enterprises, I lost touch with my earlier attitudes toward my own health. I lost a heritage of self-reliance and I drifted away from what I now recognize was a natural synthesis between healing and science. But in my forties the message was renewed for me. The free ride of youth was over, and any aberration of my lifestyle presented itself to me as an ache, or a tiredness, or an emotional gyration. Doctors didn't help much, and everyone I knew seemed to be having similar experiences. I had to recover my independence and learn again that the human body is a marvelous mechanism, which, with proper responsibility, generally heals itself.

I continued my teaching and research but began to explore many of the activities described in this book. I found I could be more responsible for my health with my own kind of holistic medicine and that my life was richer because of it.

These experiences have influenced my professional life and this book is one of the results. It combines both scholarship and personal experience in an examination of the possibility of health care for body, mind, and spirit simultaneously. Reports from many other persons on what assuming responsibility for such care is like are interwoven with my personal research and observations.

This is not a "how-to" book. After many interviews with physicians and healers of all sorts, I decided that the experiences of their patients were the most valuable message. I have blended their individual descriptions with the results of my personal inquiry.

Many people have devoted time to discussing the content of this book with me, many more than I could possibly name here. Nearly everyone I encountered wanted to share their health experiences with me. My sincere thanks to all of them.

To Shirley Leitch and Alfred French, M.D., both of whom influenced me more deeply than they have been aware of, no doubt, I wish to express a special gratitude.

Atlanta   Jack LaPatra
April 1978

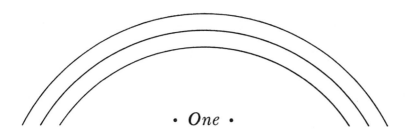

· One ·

A Return to Hippocrates

A quiet revolution is under way in American medicine and health care. Quite apart from headline-making malpractice cases and proposed national health insurance legislation, there has been a gradual transformation of health care in the United States that has been *initiated by the patients.*

Working primarily from their own perceptions, increasing numbers of patients are finding ways to blend scientific healing as practiced by modern physicians with the metaphysical healing provided by a wide variety of other practitioners. The objective—whole body healing.

What a wonderful natural concept it is, this idea that has been dubbed holistic healing. *Holism* refers to the principle in which the living organism is seen as a whole that is more than the mere sum of its interacting parts. The interdependence of all the parts critically determines the nature of the existence of the entire organism. Growing numbers of us are recognizing the deep interdependence of body, mind, emotion, and spirit, and working toward the good health of all of those simultaneously rather than separately.

The new breed of holistically-minded patient no longer

1

gives up his or her power in a passive patient-healer relationship. These patients assume increased responsibility for their own well-being by finding ways to magnify their own self-healing powers.

The consciousness of almost all Americans regarding health care is gradually changing. It's difficult to talk to almost anyone on the subject of health without eliciting a horror story from his or her medical background, and that is part of the stimulus for change.

Beginning approximately in the middle of this century, a number of American patients began to realize that the bloom was off the rose for American scientific medicine, and that doctors were not going to be able to deliver what patients expected. Too many patients had experienced too many disappointments after receiving health services.

The health consciousness of many people in earlier times, and perhaps of a majority even today, is exemplified by the following scene from a B movie or throwaway novel: In a dense African jungle a safari of Americans is attacked and captured by wild natives. The whites are taken to a village for torture or death. With their faithful bearer acting as interpreter, the Americans learn that the African chief is in a foul mood because of the serious illness of his beautiful young daughter. One member of the safari, a young, handsome doctor, steps forward, kicks aside the pagan symbols and the wildly dancing witch doctor, and pops a pill in the sick woman's mouth. Within moments the chief's daughter rises from her sick bed to embrace the doctor while the Americans bask in the chief's gratitude. As the scene closes a sumptuous party is being held as the witch doctor skulks into the jungle.

An exaggeration? Not by much. Many generations of Americans have been brought up and conditioned to believe that Western medical science is miraculous. Yet more and more of us are remembering or understanding that healing was successfully practiced for thousands of years before the availability of the relatively recent factual

2

knowledge we think of as modern medical science.

Western culture, like many other cultures throughout history, has pursued the illusion of health and happiness as a goal. We of Western culture have flown the banner of Science at the head of our particular expedition to paradise. But today, looking at health and healing cross-culturally or historically, it is apparent that alternatives to a rational scientific approach to health are available. More and more Americans are exploring those alternatives.

As a nation, our notions of medical care are a curious amalgam of fact and fantasy. One of the most pervasive ideas is that since medical care involves life or death, it takes priority over all other issues. The person who has just been hit by a train might agree; the normal newborn child with healthy ancestors, however, can live most of his or her life with little connection to physicians, and, as the infirmities of old age appear, doctors will have little to offer.

Disease is largely self-limiting and health services primarily serve to ease natural recovery. If you have an unhealthy lifestyle, you may require more complex health services, but generally when a physician intervenes, it is to reassure and then nature does the work. Rarely is life itself at stake.

Better health is frequently equated with improved medical care, but the two are far from synonymous. The doctor basically functions as a pathologist. He or she is interested in you only when you deviate from the normal. Medical school programs make the doctor essentially an anatomical detective. Competition for excellence in the medical profession centers on identifying any very rare anatomical departure from some norm—the rarer the better. If you visit physicians for counseling when you are feeling well, it's quite likely they will be bored and obliquely suggest that you are wasting their time. And you are. Their interest is in illness, not health.

If you are lucky enough to see a doctor who thinks about preventive medicine, that doctor will probably tell

3

you to eat better food, drive more slowly, smoke and drink less, avoid drugs, relax more, and the like. Most of us know these things, but many patients prefer the "repair job" to confronting the cause. One of the doctor's major functions is to enable patients to go on doing the things that are bad for them without killing themselves any sooner than is necessary.

In terms of the problems of society as a whole, doctors often ignore causality. Can you imagine a prescription being written that tries to provide something helpful for a patient experiencing poverty, decaying housing, or social alienation? Yet clearly these are causal factors in health problems.

The average life span of Americans lags substantially behind that of people in many other Western countries. Medical researchers are attempting to identify the complex causal factors behind this statistic, but the answer may be simply that we Americans tend to overeat, overdrink, and generally overindulge. Or perhaps the pace at which we work and play is killing us, along with the frustrations that persist even in the face of a high standard of living. We have been freed from our ancestors' obsession with death and disease, an obsession caused by the threats of physical danger, nutritional deficiency, and infectious fever. However, serious new threats have emerged in the form of vascular disease, cancer, and mental illness.

Perhaps the most insidious modern disease of all is boredom, which results in an overindulgence in passive forms of entertainment, loss of touch with the events of the world around us, driving around with no special place to go, meaningless vacations which we take simply because the time is available. The results of boredom range from simple escapism with drugs and alcohol to suicide.

One of the paradoxes of today's medical scene is that many Americans believe that the most direct way they can contribute to their own health is to make money available for the creation of new drugs to deal with their maladies.

4

There is inadequate general recognition that the incidence of these maladies is directly related to the lifestyle which many Americans choose. There are many chinks in our cultural armor. For instance, the American is generally well-known internationally for good humor and easy-going ways, yet one in four of our citizens will have to seek some form of mental health counseling. The correction of mismanagements of everyday life is the outstanding aim of the people who are searching for holistic healing.

Our modern culture still harbors concepts of seventeenth century scientific materialism, and any idea not in accord with this is likely to be relegated to the status of cultism. An even worse fate for an idea is for it to be labeled *occult,* that is, related to the supernatural. We will see how some of the activities of the new breed of patient have been labeled *cultism.*

Throughout the ages and all over the world it was a common illusion that the good life was identifiable with a natural life. Any straying from a lifestyle which was not close to nature was thus believed to result in illness. Early healers believed that sickness was predominately caused, not by physical factors, but by deleterious influences from the social environment ranging from poverty to excessive interest in social status. These external influences upset the natural harmony and illness followed.

It was accepted that humans had an instinct for health; that they were endowed, as a part of their birthright, with a kind of biological wisdom. We can observe today that civilized humans have apparently lost their instinct for health, and that modern medical science has not provided an appropriate replacement.

What can be credited to modern medical science? For one thing, there is no question that scientific medicine has helped to deal with the negative side effects of urban and industrial civilization. Yet to give full credit to scientific

5

medicine for stemming the tide of infectious disease over the last century is another matter. When the scientists went into action just before the turn of the twentieth century, the efforts of earlier social reformers had already reduced the effects of poor nutrition and the spread of infectious diseases. The records of those times show that the trends toward improvement were well established and medical science has not significantly altered them.

Consider the increase in life expectancy in this century. On a statistical basis, life span has been increased, but epidemiologists have shown that the increase has been due not so much to better health in the adult years of life as to the spectacular decrease in infant mortality. More children are surviving, not because of the availability of new drugs or health services, but because of better nutrition and sanitary practices. Life expectancy past the age of forty-five is only slightly greater today than several decades ago in spite of so-called scientific breakthroughs.

Let's take a look at the strategy of medical science in dealing with infectious diseases. Hygienic practices are combined with immunization and antimicrobial drugs to thwart and destroy microbes. There are often irritating side effects from the drugs and the microbes frequently return with greater resistance to the drugs. A measure of control is achieved, however.

What about alternatives to this approach? The biologist offers a natural alternative. He points out that animals and plants, as well as humans, can live peacefully with their most notorious microbial enemies. A generation ago there was almost daily contact between people and the tubercle bacillus. Many people became a little tuberculous, but the flow of normal creative life was not interrupted for them. There was no vaccine, and whether the illness was slight or serious, there was little medicine could do.

Each year, before polio innoculations were available, millions of young people were infected by exposure to polio virus, but of those it was only several thousand who actually experienced the disease poliomyelitis. The selection mechanism of polio is not known. It is obvious, however, that this crippling disease requires more than just the invading virus.

When Louis Pasteur proposed his germ theory, he did not visualize a simplistic connection between germs and disease. Many Americans, because they lack education or have been miseducated by oversimplifying physicians, believe that germs cause disease, and that the way to deal with germs is to kill them with drugs. Pasteur pointed out that the response of the germ-infected individual is determined by hereditary factors, nutritional state, environment, including climate, and mental state.

Scientific medicine in general and the germ theory in particular are given too much credit for the improvement of the general health of people. Our memories are very short when we give credit for the control of infectious diseases to the widespread use of antibacterial drugs. A review of medical history shows that increased control of infectious disease is a trend that extends through all of recorded history. The antibiotics of recent times would not cause even a small blip on the chart. Rene Dubos has pointed out that the introduction of easy-to-launder, inexpensive cotton undergarments and of transparent glass that brought light into the most humble dwelling have contributed more to the control of infection than all drugs and medical practices combined.

Illness causality is extremely complex and not well understood. Is the characteristic microbe of a disease a symptom rather than a cause? That question will not be answered by this book, but it is important to know that the question exists and remains unanswered.

In spite of scientific principles that seemingly emphasize causality, it is extremely rare for a complete account of the causation of a disease to be given by modern medicine. National efforts to determine the causes of cancer, arteriosclerosis, and mental disorders can only be described as

7

frenetic. Causality for these and other major medical problems of our times remains undiscovered.

If we assume that disease is not the direct outcome of a single determinant factor, the opposite position may make the search for disease causality by the laboratory scientist a hopeless pursuit. Most researchers would agree today that disease states are the *indirect* outcome of an *array* of conditions. The search for these physical, economic, social, and emotional conditions and their indirect effects is an incredibly difficult scientific task.

Sometimes, but not often, the search for disease causality has led to ways of controlling the disease. Despite such added knowledge, however, the cause of the disease remains obscure. Although we put out a fire with water, few fires are caused by a lack of water. An example of the lack of connection between cause and control is the treatment of diabetes in humans. The discovery of insulin, which controls diabetes, was a magnificent scientific contribution; however, the causality of diabetes is still far from clear.

Detecting causality from control methods is hopeless when relief is achieved by a substance which doesn't even occur in the body. An obvious example is aspirin, a synthetic drug that is foreign to the body and can demonstrably ease aches and pains. Although the problem of determining disease causality has frustrated healers since antiquity (ancient physicians observed that the severity and prevalence of many diseases varied according to geographical locations, social customs, and economic levels of people), the concept of causality implies the logical approach of modern science; but, in fact, prior to the late nineteenth century causality had little to do with scientific medical thought. A state of health was considered to be an equilibrium among man, his environment, and the various forces at work in the body. Disease occurred when the equilibrium was disturbed. Disharmony for the Navajos was the thwarting of their wish to live "in accord with the mountain soil, the pollen of all the plants, and other sacred things."

Medical science has been able to establish that causality depends on the past in two ways. Both genetic differences and past experiences of individuals have the effect of making one man's meat another man's poison. The Greeks have given us the word *allergy* to label one of the many ways in which past experience influences an individual's response today.

Harmony with nature and within ourselves is an intuitively attractive idea for all times. Flowing, fitting in with, or going along with the natural forces of life makes a great deal of common sense. The idea that harmony with the world around you leads to living wisely has been a recurring philosophical theme. Yet today people generally find it easier to depend on healers than to attempt the more difficult task of living wisely. It seems our culture has conditioned us to a state of disharmony rather than harmony.

Dr. Irving Oyle, a well-known medical writer, calls attention to a cardiology conference where it was reported that an excessive number of patients are choosing to have coronary bypass operations for early symptoms of heart trouble rather than modifying the lifestyle that eventually leads to coronary disease. And so a quick cure via a risky operation is preferred to giving up smoking, slowing down, or losing weight. For many, bed confinement in a hospital following an illness is more unsettling than the possibility of delayed physical recovery caused by premature release from the hospital.

We have all heard of the Hippocratic oath, which physicians honor by tradition; but how many people, including physicians, have read any of the other writings of Hippocrates? Hippocratic writings are to medicine what the Bible is to literature. Fitness to the environment is essential for health in the Hippocratic view. When changes in conditions

9

are too abrupt to allow natural adaptive mechanisms to function, disease follows. The true Hippocratic tradition emphasizes the whole patient and his relationship to his environment.

The germ theory and the limited causality concepts of scientific medicine have broken the spell of the Hippocratic tradition for almost a century. Hippocrates believed that the sick body triggers natural forces to restore equilibrium and to recover good health. The knowledge of his time was so limited that the corrective mechanisms were not known or understood, but the basic idea was clear. The physician was to intervene only in the most natural way. Another foundation of Hippocratic thought was the notion that humans have a good chance of avoiding disease if they live reasonably. Physicians were useful only for wounds and epidemics.

The word *physician* comes from the Greek word meaning *nature*. Hippocrates wrote that a healer "must be skilled in Nature and must strive to know what man is in relation to food, drink, occupation, and which effect each of these has on the other." Working from these concepts Hippocrates achieved an unimpeachable reputation as the greatest healer of his time. In all cultures and at all times in world history there have been remarkable healers. Successful healing did not begin with modern scientific medicine.

In retrospect, it is apparent that many successful healers of the past learned through experience to manipulate empirically the psychological, physiological, and social factors that affected the health of their patients.

The Hippocratic concept of healing has far-ranging implications. For example, the sickness of an individual is not easily separated from the sickness of society. Causality is extremely complex, but the connection cannot be denied. In our own time it is likely that the stresses and frustrations of the Vietnam War contributed to a great deal of illness in this country.

Any profound change in social patterns influences the

10

health of nations and the incidence of disease in their populations. Although it's difficult to prove statistically because much time must pass and several generations must be studied, such diverse factors as the shortening of working hours, the refinement of food products, and the sophistication of medical practices surely affect the health of large populations.

What we know now about health and disease appears to be superficial. There are powerful long-term forces about which we know little that affect the health trends of large populations. We have yet to discover the fundamental physical and biological laws of the world that are the basis of the most deeply-rooted habits and beliefs of humankind. In the absence of specific knowledge and with increasing distrust of the value of the knowledge that is available, many Americans are finding their own ways to improve and sustain their own health. Their changes in personal health styles and quests are responses to the failure of modern health and medical services to meet modern man's needs.

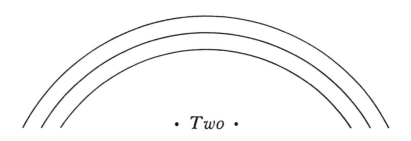

· *Two* ·

The Healer's Ritual

When we want to visit a doctor and don't know one, information is more difficult to locate than when we are buying a new car, planning a cruise to the South Seas, or selecting a restaurant for a special evening out. There is no consumer's guide to physicians.

American doctors are generally well trained. They attend good schools and receive accreditation from states, specialty boards, and the like. By custom or by law they display their credentials in their offices. Those documents may tell you something about the doctor's professional background, but what do you know—really know—about the person you choose to heal you? An ill person looking in the yellow pages of the telephone book or inquiring of a friend in trying to locate a doctor doesn't know how to assess the various physicians' qualifications.

It doesn't seem appropriate to ask the fee for diagnosing a generally rundown feeling. Even when the malady is more specific, what patient is willing and able to ask a series of doctors, "What does it cost to repair a broken finger, and will the finger be perfectly normal afterwards?"

Even after a seemingly adequate physician has been located, the information flow can be a trickle. Though doctors are discouraged from publishing information about their training or practice by state laws against professional advertising, they bear partial responsibility for continuing to foster and cherish mystery in medicine. Think of the prescription written in hieroglyphics and the enigmatic smile after the blood pressure has been taken. Or the nurse's stolid mask and heavy silence after the reading of the thermometer.

I have a friend who, with little encouragement, will tell the story of her young daughter's visit to a hospital for minor surgery. Annie had been observed, tested, and medicated for weeks before a specialist finally pinpointed the difficulty and called to say that she should be at the hospital at 7:00 AM on a certain day. Annie's mother was exasperated to tears by the exchange with the physician that followed. To get any picture of what was about to happen, she had to interrogate the resisting doctor with questions like these:

"What hospital?"

"Where in the hospital?"

"How long will Annie be there?"

"How can I help?"

"What is going to happen?"

"Will there by any pain involved?"

"Will there be a difficult aftermath?"

"What are the dangers?"

The main issue was that Annie was very frightened of doctors because of earlier traumatic contacts. Her mother's role was to comfort her and boost her confidence, but it had to be done in an atmosphere of evasion and jargon-laden explanation. Overlaying the entire process was the parent's requirement of complete honesty to Annie.

It is true that some procedures and conventions have been established for the convenience and protection of doctors; but often the effect of such conventions is to humble the patient. Though this may be necessary to make patients manageable or even tolerable, it is a risky business. Most patients fear to some degree, not death necessarily, but almost always incapacity or destitution. Research has demonstrated that the most critical ingredient in the recovery of a sick person is *belief*. The patient must believe in his or her own capacity for getting well and in the value of the healing technique. It is difficult for the patient's belief to be fostered by professional behavior that creates a gulf between the healer and the patient.

Contemporary medicine, like ancient medicine, is based upon a humane interaction between a sufferer and a healer, upon a trusting personal relationship between a physician and a patient. Most people consult lawyers only at rare intervals. Students may see their teachers regularly, but generally they have little individual contact with them. Many persons have no contact with clergymen from one year to the next. However, it is a rare person who does not seek the services of a doctor at least once a year.

The transaction with a doctor is but one ingredient in a long process that begins with a person *perceiving* that something is awry. The process culminates ideally with the person experiencing a mental sense, a body sense, and a social sense of complete well-being.

It may be enlightening to follow the sickness rituals of an American and an African who become ill and see how they interact with their respective healing systems. As we will see, there are superficial differences between the experiences of the American and the African; but there are also incredible similarities, especially with respect to mystery and ritual. Think of the American as yourself. Let's look first at activities and options.

The beginning of an illness is often very fuzzy. You may wake up in the morning with a vague sense of uneasiness, a faint suggestion that something is amiss. Unusual sensations occur that don't change the activities of your day but generate plaintive remarks such as, "I'm not up to par today," or "Is there something going around?" If you're

14

the stoical type, you may suppress all of this and proceed with business as usual.

When more specific things like twinges of pain or sluggishness follow, your outward behavior begins to change and the people around you may start saying, "You don't seem to be yourself today." Now you're beginning to admit to yourself that you're sick. Not a big deal. But sick. Perhaps your body aches in every joint and your throat is scratchy. No appetite. Maybe that familiar instrument from your youth, the thermometer, declares you have a fever.

At this stage you may take some aspirin, but in doing so you get a warning from Washington: the Food and Drug Administration, an agent of the federal government, announces on the label of the aspirin bottle, "In case of persistent fever, call your doctor." Bad tidings are coming to you from both within and without.

There is no doubt that you are getting sick. What to do about it? The options are many. The choice might be to see a minister or friend, read a book, or visit a health food store. Or diet, exercise, and pray. Or just wait. You may know that about three-quarters of all ailments go away by themselves under fair conditions. But what if you fear that you are in the other quarter?

You can delay action and hope for the best. You can visit an establishment or a location that provides a helpful service. You can purchase an appliance or other equipment for treating the difficulty. You can obtain a nonprescription drug at the pharmacy or use home remedies. You can re-examine your whole regimen and follow healthier procedures. And finally, after you have exhausted your own resources, you can consult a physician, either in your home or at his office.

I want to emphasize how much decision-making power the sick person has, so let's look at the range of choices within each of these larger options.

If you don't want to just wait you can visit a service

establishment that might help. You might try a weight-reducing salon or a Turkish bath. Steam baths attempt to "purify" the body with heavy sweating, which drains away body poisons. Hot mineral baths at spas are believed to be curative and rejuvenating. Clinics featuring high colonic irrigations are available, and many Americans fly to dry Arizona or sunny Florida for their "healthy" climates. Some of our more athletic citizens work out at gymnasiums to set themselves right.

As for appliances or equipment, there are many. There are sun lamps, hot water bottles, enema tubes, trusses, chin straps, vaporizers, atomizers, heating pads, elastic bandages, foot baths, vibrators, and exercise machines. You may choose any of these devices to reduce your discomfort.

There are also many over-the-counter drugs available. Gone are the days of the traveling medicine man who sold a single concoction that would relieve aches and pains, cure snake bites, remove warts, restore "manly vigor," and grow hair on your head. Today you can choose from an enormous variety of specialized tonics and preparations at your local drugstore.

If you believe in home remedies, you can take a home-made cough syrup derived from onions boiled slowly and mixed with sugar or honey. Sulphur and molasses are still used today to thin the blood. Many a cold is attacked with whiskey and hot lemonade. A salt water gargle relieves a sore throat and a raw piece of beef may take care of a black eye. A reliable laxative is lemon juice and hot water first thing in the morning.

The next choice open to you is to pursue anything that will be beneficial to your general health or reduce any specific discomfort. Soak in the sun, get a good-looking tan, and build up resistance to disease. Change your lifestyle to a spartan mode with plenty of cold showers and open windows at night: do vigorous deep breathing at regular periods during the day. Fast, or become a vege-

16

tarian. Follow the formulas disclosed by old people when asked the secret of their longevity, such as abstinence from tobacco or alcohol, a shot of whiskey before supper, regular exercise or the lack of it, or a teaspoonful of baking soda after every meal.

The important thing to remember about the options is that *the choice is up to you.* After considering a multitude of personal and environmental factors, the person experiencing the distressing symptoms will decide what to do. Our medical industry is an illness system and generally *we* decide whether or not to inject ourselves into it.

Let's assume that eventually you do decide to see a traditional doctor. Several questions must be answered first. Do you want to see a general practitioner or one of the many specialists available? How can you identify the particular physician you want to see? How will you know if his qualifications and skills are superior or even adequate? And beyond these questions, you may ask: Can you afford the services of this particular physician?

If your problem is mental, the task of deciding which type of therapy will be most successful is even more complex. This is assuming, of course, that you are willing to risk the possibility of being labeled *crazy.*

Though it is rare nowadays, let's say that a physician has been located and has agreed to make a house call. The doctor arrives in a car, generally a large, dark car, and the odds are high that the doctor is male. His car has the M.D. license plate and the Aesculapian emblem—the one with the snakes. It's likely that the car is festooned with other stickers and labels which grant admittance and parking at various health facilities, restricted housing areas, and country or tennis clubs. There's a fair chance that there is an A.O.P.A. (Aircraft Owners and Pilots' Association) sticker in the window.

The doctor is almost always well-dressed and maybe even dapper. You can tell a lot about where he lives by the style of his clothes—country tweedy, city sophisticate, or

17

suburban sport. His manner may be jovial, deadpan, or even deferential, but your response is based mainly on the sense that the person walking from the curb to the house represents all the power of western medicine, and you are a westerner. This perception, coupled with the typical patient's fear of being ill, makes the interaction that follows incredibly complex on every level.

The doctor's symbol of authority is his black bag. It is well known in medical circles that the smaller the bag the larger the fees are likely to be.

The recitation of symptoms doesn't take you too long, and it seems apparent that he's heard all that before. He takes your temperature and pulse, looks at your eyes, listens here and there with his stethoscope, and then four years of college, four more of medical school, a year or two of internship, and maybe three more of residency qualify him to utter sympathetically, "It's a virus. It's been going around."

Let's step back a moment and take a closer look at what is happening. The next chapter will consider the point more carefully, but I want to emphasize here that attitudes towards healing in America are essentially outgrowths of technological civilization. Our medicine is characterized by impersonal relations, procedures unfamiliar to the lay person, passive roles of patient and relatives, and general control of the situation by professional healers.

Doctors are among those people in our society whose roles continuously expose them to the unhappy side of life. Motorcycle cops, police court magistrates, hotel clerks, divorce lawyers, call girls, customs officers, credit managers, department store detectives, headwaiters, bartenders, and cashiers are among others who incessantly hear complaints, excuses, evasions, rationalizations, and just plain self-serving lies. Can you imagine the boredom, or worse, the depression, of listening to the same negative stories day after day? The development of the wooden face and the fishy eye are inevitable—except for doctors,

18

therapists, and nurses. These health professionals have taken an oath that they won't be bored. Nevertheless, human failings, or the need for some kind of emotional detachment, often give the doctor a cold, impersonal demeanor.

In the typical transaction with the doctor the patient gives up his or her personal powers and strengths almost totally and is in the control, and sometimes at the mercy, of the doctor. Haven't you ever felt helpless in that moment when a physician fixes a stern gaze on you and in an authoritarian voice instructs you what to do next with yourself? Each day more Americans are sensing the danger of such doctor-patient roles.

Returning now to your virus and the doctor's visit, note that phase one of the doctor-patient ritual has been completed. A rational, scientifically based diagnosis has been made. In phase two, if the doctor is of the new school in which mystery is minimized, he will probably tell you that the virus is a self-limiting disease and that you will be better in a few days. He is likely to follow that by saying, "Just to make sure, I'll give you a prescription." In your passive, powerless position you are not likely to question the logic of that statement. In fact, every discernable signal from the doctor is carefully monitored by you in silence. You study his every facial expression, nuance of voice, and movement of body to help ameliorate the fear that gnaws at you when you are sick.

The last phase of the doctor's home visit involves his making a note of the charge and requesting a call at a certain time if you are not better. This request shows his concern, helps in case of a malpractice claim, and adds a little uncertainty to your conviction that the diagnosis is correct.

Before considering what happens after the doctor's visit, let's review the more common instance of the patient visiting the doctor's office. An appointment at a mutually appropriate time must be arranged and you must get to the doctor's waiting room. If no appointment is necessary, you may be assailed by doubts even more overwhelming than the discomfort of waiting while sick for an appointment with a busy doctor. Surely the doctor cannot be competent if there is no appointment schedule.

The waiting room, like most parts of the doctor's office, exudes tradition. Waiting rooms seem to be all the same. The ambiance is uncertain, and the people, silent and inscrutable, glance with feigned interest at the illustrations in outdated periodicals. The chairs are uncomfortable and the occupants appear dedicated to concealing their own mysterious illnesses. At one end of the waiting room, probably in a glass fortress, is the receptionist, who tries to combine total loyalty to "the Doctor" and personal benefaction (at a distance) to the patients.

If this is your first visit, part of the ritual is the collection of vital statistics, including the name of your health insurance carrier and your Social Security number. You may also be asked to fill out a health history sheet. While waiting for your inevitably late appointment with the doctor, a look around at others who are waiting confirms your wisdom in planning to see this particular physician. The doctor can't lose in this assessment. If the patients look upper-class, you figure the doctor must be good, but if they appear to be ordinary working people, you are impressed by his democratic spirit and love for humanity.

When your name is called you may be sent directly to the examination room, or you may begin by talking to the doctor in his office. After reviewing your history with him and talking over your complaints you go to the examination room, where you struggle with the examination gown. Is it meant to be open in front or back? In either case it's a humiliating costume. The examination room has all the trappings of a modern practice: scales and gauges of one sort or another, bottles, phials, dishes, balls of cotton, a syringe lying casually upon a desk, and an examination couch with an ugly disposable paper cover.

The doctor proceeds with the examination even though

20

he is already pretty sure of what ails you and what he's going to do about it. He figures you won't believe him without an examination. Typically, your body orifices are examined in various ways, body parts are pressed and tapped, and the stethoscope is used liberally. It is common for doctors to omit palpation, a form of laying on of hands, if it does not seem necessary for the diagnosis. This omission has given birth to the image of the doctor who never touches his patient. The reassuring touch of a caring physician has more potential healing power than medical school ever suggested.

The examination is a ritual, both for the patient and for the doctor. The doctor may not be sure of the rationale for what he is doing, and he may rush; but he does believe that what he is doing is important because it is within the patient's expectations. At some point in your visit, the doctor is likely to glance at your medical records, quote the date of your last physical examination; and make a casual pitch for its annual repetition. More ritual. Sure, the annual physical examination is a good income source for the doctor, but there is growing agreement among health professionals that by its nature and brevity the typical annual examination is of little benefit to the patient.

In most other professions the collecting of data is followed by a period of time for analysis, but generally it is part of the medical ritual that the doctor be immediately ready with his diagnosis. His well-meaning attempt to speed the process increases the chance of error in diagnosis.

Now let's think back to the doctor's home visit, where we left off with his diagnosis of a virus-caused illness. Assume the same diagnosis has just been delivered in the doctor's office, and the same prescription rendered.

In the case of virus, the prescription is likely to be one of three drugs: an antibiotic, an analgesic, or an antihistamine. Antibiotics have been shown to have no value in curing a virus, and aspirin is a safer and cheaper analgesic

21

than the multi-colored capsules obtained from the pharmacy with the prescription. Antihistamines often interfere with the body's response to infection and are potentially dangerous to children, pregnant women, and the aged. So although the prescription part of the healing ritual has been indulged, the payoff seems uncertain.

In next to no time at all you are back out on the street again, already feeling considerably more relaxed. In fact, while you were just sitting in the waiting room, the symptoms seemed to have eased.

Following your visit to the doctor, you are back in the decision-making seat again, especially if there is no follow-up visit. A decision must be made about the effort you will make to follow the doctor's instructions. Will the drugs be purchased and taken exactly as prescribed? Will rest periods be observed even if absence from work is necessary? Finally, you must decide when the symptoms are gone and the label *well person* is appropriate. And does *well* mean complete physiological, psychological, and sociological wellness, or will you settle for less?

Almost all of us have experienced the process just described. The reason for reviewing the act of seeing a doctor is to emphasize that the patient's activities begin long before the physical confrontation with the doctor and continue for some time after. The patient's behavior and decision-making in all phases of this process depend on a myriad of factors, including social status, past conditioning, and personal characteristics.

In the United States we do not emphasize preventive medical care as is done in England. Therefore, the burden is ours to determine whether or not we will seek a healer. It is unlikely that a professional will help us with this decision.

The fundamental ingredients in the process of seeing a doctor are: the perception of discomfort, awareness of the body, the personal attitude towards health and healing,

22

and the health payoff expected from a healing ritual. The critical thread connecting these fundamentals is our sensitivity to our own feelings, both physical and emotional.

The ability to observe or perceive the changes that occur when we get sick varies enormously from person to person. Ours is not generally a "body-oriented" culture. Status in our society does not depend on the condition of a person's body. Instead, the emphasis is on income, power, and intellect.

A body-oriented person is capable of detecting almost immediately a minor rash on the back of a knee, or slightly heavier breathing after climbing stairs. Another person may require dramatic body symptoms like fainting before noticing anything.

Many of us do not perceive symptoms that are not obviously visible. How in tune with your body are you? Are you aware of the constant stream of messages being sent by your body to keep you informed of how well it's doing? Not many of us are perceptive to the extent that we could be. Some researchers speculate that with proper training we could focus our attention on individual cells of our bodies.

The foregoing description of getting sick and seeing a doctor in America is familiar to us all, but there can be much more variation in that process than most of us realize. A way of beginning to explore the potential variations is to compare seeing a doctor in our culture with seeing a healer in another culture. Let's construct a composite healing process which a black man somewhere in Africa conceivably might experience.

The African awakens one morning with confusing sensations of general discomfort. At the outset he sends for one of his wives from her quarters in the family compound and she is told to collect the leaves of a particular plant which grows in profusion in a nearby meadow. These leaves, steeped in a large pot of boiling water, provide a tea which is known to be helpful for his particular malaise. He drinks a large gourd of the tea, and to maximize the effect of the medicine, he washes in the tea while chanting healing rhymes.

Waiting for some relief, he sprawls listlessly on a bench in front of his hut to greet his friends who pass his door. There is no withdrawal or secrecy about his discomfort. When friends inquire about his health, he describes his indisposition in detail, and they reply with elaborate condolences and advice regarding healing herbs, witch doctors, and herbalists whose services are known to be excellent.

Later in the day a messenger is sent with a request for the witch doctor to call. The witch doctor is a highly respected member of the community who has attained his envied position by long years of study and apprenticeship to a successful witch doctor. He appears wearing a mask and a feathered headress and carrying the tools of his trade in a bag. He is considered qualified to deal with diseases caused by external malevolent forces or those thought to be the result of the patient's own bad deeds.

The witch doctor assesses the worth of the possessions in his patient's home so that he can ask a fee commensurate with his patient's status. Then he asks questions like, "What taboos have you broken? Have you had a fight with a friend? Have you had any bad dreams?"

From his medical bag, which contains stones, bones, beads, paints, shells, herbs, and parts of animals, he may take chicken bones and make a diagnosis by casting the bones and studying the patterns. He might prick the sick man's skin with a thorn and observe the response. While the witch doctor forms his diagnosis, the family pleads with him for his best efforts.

The witch doctor's therapy comes in many forms. He chants, sings, and dances while shaking a rattle. He burns strange substances to banish evil spirits. He lets blood to eliminate poisons from the sick man. He makes mystical symbols with root ink on a piece of bark which the patient

24

then chews and swallows. The witch doctor's healing efforts are vigorous, blatant, and visible. Intense personal energy flows from him to his patient.

At last, exhausted by his labors, the witch doctor rests and accepts the grateful attention of the family. Food and drink are brought. His departure is usually marked by long and complicated instructions for further treatment.

The analogy to our culture must be obvious. The behavior of the physician and the witch doctor is largely ritualistic and designed to meet the expectations of the patients. Both patients act out their sickness roles in a manner appropriate for the particular healer. It is as if the healer and the sick person are actors in a drama that facilititates the release of the natural healing powers of the body.

Very little is known about the relationship between symptoms, the therapy of the healer, and the patient's recovery. As Lester Breslow, Dean of the U.C.L.A. School of Public Health has stated, "Some medical care is good for you, a great deal is irrelevant, and unfortunately, some of it is harmful." My own experience and observation lead me to estimate that ten per cent of medical therapy is helpful in curing illness (not just alleviating symptoms), eighty per cent is irrelevant, and ten per cent may be harmful.

To carry our healing example a bit further, let's assume that the sick African decides to visit a herbalist to guarantee his cure. In the early evening, dressed with care against the cooler night air, the sick man and several younger male companions proceed to the home of the chosen herbal healer.

The healer's consulting room also serves as his bedroom and living room. Above the door is a protective charm. In the corner of the room is a shrine with a carved wooden figure and offerings of scraps of food. In every part of the room there are collections of medical materials—seeds on a scrap of paper, black ointment in a cracked earthenware pot. Various powders are stored in every imaginable container. Bundles of dried plants are strewn everywhere. Unidentifiable parts of small animals hang drying from the ceiling.

In a discussion with the herbalist the focus is not on the patient's symptoms, but rather on the particular circumstances and time at which they were observed to have begun. Perhaps the symptoms began in such a way that the patient was prevented from attending to a business matter, or the symptoms arose after an argument with a friend.

A special combination of ingredients is formed in a very careful sequence to the accompaniment of a special incantation. The proper time to take the potion is rigorously specified, and there are usually prohibitions regarding the patient's diet or behavior while being treated by the healer.

The sick man returns home with his expectations completely fulfilled and he is ready to begin to feel well again. If the symptoms persist, there are many possible explanations within this healing system. The potion may not have been powerful enough or a vital ingredient of the remedy was missing or debased. For example, the eye of a rare mammal. The accompanying chanting may not have been pronounced correctly. Or it is possible that some other person, wishing the patient no good, had been simultaneously consulting another herbalist to have a countermedicine prepared.

The sick man may decide that a more powerful healer is required. He might consult an elderly, wise priest whose healing techniques involve elaborate sacrifices and consultations with gods which, if successful, would cause a fundamental reorganization of the sick man's personal relationships and plans.

It is clear that the American and the African of the preceding narratives experience medical situations with many superficial differences. In both cases, however, the healer and his patient share a common language and the same basic ideas for discussing illness. In both societies the sickness behavior of the ill person is predictable.

A useful classification of illness in any society requires four general categories: minor illnesses, which are self-limiting; chronic illnesses, which are marked by an uneven succession of partial recoveries, with times when the patient feels well and relapses when the uncomfortable symptoms return; symptoms that are produced in people who are anxious or upset for a variety of reasons; and acute conditions, which may involve severe infections, surgical emergencies, and dangerous diseases.

The first three categories, short-term minor illnesses, chronic complaints, and illnesses with a psychological basis, are all likely to benefit from interaction with *any* healer. The first type is self-limited. Chronic conditions, the second type, fluctuate and symptoms can be alleviated. For the anxious patient with the third type of malady, understanding, reassurance, and help with personal problems are needed.

If we compare the African healing system to the American medical system, we can speculate that the African healer does well with the first three types of illnesses, and the American (or western) doctor with the first two and the fourth. Western medicine is clearly superior in the treatment of acute conditions, while African healers are of better service to patients with personal, emotional, and social disturbances. Most other sickness is dealt with by the body, and whatever healing technique has been used, in whatever society, is given credit. In neither the American nor the African medical setting are there a sufficient number of conspicuous failures to raise serious doubts about the value of the existing arrangements or to challenge belief in the system itself. It is clear, however, that there is more than one way to facilitate the healing process.

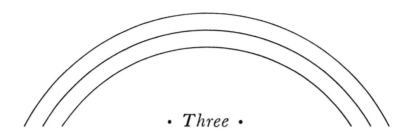

· *Three* ·

Metaphysical Healing

Holistic healing is a marvelously intriguing concept. The term has already captivated the media and become a staple, trendy conversation piece. However, scientific medicine has not yet accumulated the requisite knowledge to allow our physicians to practice holistic healing. The doctor is often in quicksand when he or she tries to answer our personal questions or respond to our varied medical needs. Intellectually, the doctor knows that healing the whole person means the *simultaneous* healing of body, mind, emotions, and spirit. Yet to speak of a person as being a *mosiac* of body, mind, emotions, and spirit, as researchers often do, is inadequate and inaccurate. Because it is an approximation of reality, such a four-part model of man is still a familiar and helpful form.

Healing itself has basically remained the same for millennia. Healers try to restore harmony in the *person*. Harmony is such a perfect word in this context; it connotes order, balance, and pleasing arrangements of our total person. It also means living in accord with nature. Continuing with this kind of imagery, we can say disease is caused by an insult to the body. Some healers merely try to restore harmony to the *body*.

In the study of health there are few details on which everyone will agree. If we accept for present purposes the provocative notion of individual harmony, including its being an intuitive rather than an intellectual idea, we have a useful basis for comparing the activities of different healers, and for examining how successfully various healers promote harmony in their patients. No matter the time or location, a sick person always seeks out in himself, or in another person or many people, the means for making himself whole and harmonious again.

In the preceding chapter we saw examples of the two major types of healing, scientific healing and metaphysical healing. The traditional physician is a scientific healer. For him, body disturbances stem from microbes, viruses, and other tiny invaders; from variations in hormones and metabolism; and from physical trauma. The scientific healer functions after illness has occurred, emphasizes symptom reduction, and often treats each illness as an isolated episode. He heals by applying allopathic therapy, which is based on a notion so simple and commonsensical that few question it. When the functioning of the body deviates from the normal, a counteracting procedure or agent is applied. If the patient is feverish, ways are found to cool him; if his blood pressure is high, it is lowered by some means. We will take a more detailed look at allopathy in the next section.

The natural sciences provide the foundation for scientific healing, which is practical and empirical and places major emphasis on the healing properties of material agents. Over a long history, various chemicals and techniques within the allopathic theme are tried. Those that succeed persist in usage. Cause and effect are often unknown, especially in the early stages of usage of a drug.

The metaphysical healer envisions himself as either the source of healing power, or as an instrument acting on behalf of some higher healing power. The faith healer does not heal, but instead provides a channel through which

29

healing powers from a divine force flow to the sick person. On the other hand, psychic healers, shamans, and sorcerers believe that they have the ability to tap deep levels of curative power in themselves. These healers often speak of having "a gift" or being among "the chosen." Metaphysical healing is founded on spiritual beliefs. Its varied practitioners frequently emphasize the unknowable character of healing.

The two types of healing appear to have nothing in common. They do overlap, however. Various materials, plants, and chemicals have been used by metaphysicians. In ancient Egypt, for one example, healers used excreta from pelicans, crocodiles, and gazelles to treat eye infections. Concoctions based on these repulsive ingredients were intended to remove or repel demons. Only recently has it been learned that these foul potions contained antibiotic substances.

Healing with placebos, psychosomatic medicine, and psychotherapy doesn't fit neatly into either of our categories, but our division of healing into two parts, though admittedly oversimplified, is still useful at this point. And we will look at these other topics in more detail later.

Spontaneous remission is a phenomenon that is neither scientific nor metaphysical, and therefore also falls outside my categories. Throughout the history of humankind, sudden, unexplained healings of nearly every kind of illness have occurred. Unquestionably, a vastly successful healer would be one whose talents justified the title "Doctor of Spontaneous Remissions." Generally, spontaneous remission does not relate to contemporary understanding of the body or its functioning or how it should be healed. The healing simply occurs, and it may be declared a miracle or a healer may attempt to take credit for the cure.

If we look at the United States from the viewpoint of the ideas in this chapter so far, we will see that scientific medicine and metaphysical healing have coexisted for a long time. Local health-belief systems and folk healers abound in all parts of this country. Furthermore, because of economic and environmental conditions and social stresses, the variety of healing activities is proliferating.

Pentacostal churches, snake handling cults, and revivalist meetings are examples of American metaphysical healing derived from Christianity. Healing evangelists such as Kathryn Kuhlman, Oral Roberts, and Billy Graham believe that they are instruments for focusing the power of God and releasing the natural healing power of the individual.

The Church of Christ, Scientist, takes the position that disease is a material illusion. Belief in a personal and helpful God is the church's basis of healing. Members of the church facilitate healing by helping the sick person overcome any "sick beliefs."

A healing belief system called *espiritismo* has widespread acceptance among Puerto Ricans, Cubans, Mexicans, and other Latin Americans in this country. The essential notion of this system is that there is an invisible world populated by spirits who can communicate with the living. The healing offered by the *expiritistas* has been studied by psychologists and psychiatrists and there is some agreement among them about its positive effect.

Many Mexican Americans believe in a concept of disease that might be called the "hot-cold" theory, and which came originally from Spain and Portugal. The central idea of this theory is that a healthy person is a suitable combination of hot and cold components. Illness results from an imbalance so that the sick person is either hot or cold. An array of foods and medicines, each with hot or cold attributes, are administered until balance is restored. There is obviously a conceptual tie to the allopathy of scientific medicine.

Many ways of looking at health in this country stem from African influences. African sorcery in one form or another, including hexing and the removal of spells, still exists in many black communities. Middle class Americans

31

who do not venture outside their own traditional beliefs may think that hexing, spells, black magic, and voodoo exist only in motion pictures or on television. However, priests of Haitian voodoo are doing healing rituals in black sections of New York City today.

There has been a wave of interest in recent years in the American Indian and in Indian healing practices. Navajo healers have received perhaps the most attention. A talk at a psychiatric conference in 1972 even described a present-day school for Navajo medicine men. The Navajos have their medical specialists, too. There are herbalists, shaman diagnosticians who use hand trembling, crystal gazing, or stargazing to determine the nature and cause of an illness; and singers who do the work of healing.

These examples are only a few of the metaphysical healing systems that exist side by side with scientific medicine. The American who pays health insurance premiums regularly and sees a doctor occasionally may be tempted to dismiss metaphysical healing as strange, and wonder why it even continues in modern times.

We will see as we go whether it is strange; and there are at least seven reasons why metaphysical healing exists and persists.

1. In any country or region where there is rapid industrialization or uneven economic development, metaphysical medicine will be found simultaneously with scientific medicine. In Brazil, where industrialization has been chaotic, highly technical medical practice is found amid many forms of metaphysical healing.

Czechoslovakia's early industrial development was concentrated in some geographic sections while others remained agricultural and at a much lower level of social development. This resulted in 1948 in a clash between mandatory, enforced scientific medical care and the traditional healing practices of the farmers.

The psychic surgeons of the Phillipine Islands, who operate with their bare hands without surgical instruments, function in the economically depressed and socially retarded (to Western eyes) back country of the islands, far from urban centers.

In the United States industrialization and urbanization have left behind many small towns and rural areas, especially in the South, Midwest, and West, where metaphysical healing ideas, unsophisticated to the city dweller, continue to flourish.

2. Immigration brings alternative healing styles into new settings. For example, thousands of Cubans who now live in New York City and Florida brought with them from Cuba an Afro-Cuban health system and religion called *santeria.*

3. The poor in developed nations often do not have access to modern health care, so alternatives are necessary, even preferred. Exiles, poor immigrants, and socially and economically oppressed minority groups frequently have health cultures that are not used by or even known to the dominant culture.

4. Any country in which modern medical care is largely unavailable or of dubious quality will have highly-evolved alternative healing systems. Certainly India and many African nations are examples; and, to a lesser extent, even the United States is moving into this category. A number of factors, among them the cost, the unavailability, and the lack of quality of traditional medicine, are causing a growing number of Americans to seek or develop alternative healing.

5. Many people choose metaphysical healing when orthodox medicine apparently fails them. The terminal cancer patient and the individual who is undergoing severe psychological stress are prime candidates. The religious flavor of the metaphysical viewpoint offers an anguished person spiritual and psychological support, which he would not normally receive in a hospital setting.

6. As modern life becomes increasingly impersonal and technological, many people gravitate toward the warmth

and spirit of metaphysical healing. They bubble with stories about their psychic readings, acupuncture treatments, or most recent horoscopes. Some individuals are continuously intrigued by the metaphysical, mystical, and occult. They want to experience everything unusual that comes along.

7. There has been a recent dramatic change in the consciousness and the value structure of the younger generation in the United States and other countries with high technological development. For these people, progressive alienation from the mainstream of culture has led to the formation of a counterculture with an incredible range of alternative lifestyles, including experimentation with metaphysical healing methods. The younger generation's attitudes have been infectious and many older persons have begun to share their interests in philosophy, oriental and other ancient cultures, and various religions and cults. In the late 1970s this "new consciousness" cuts across all social classes and educational levels.

A friend of mine lived in a commune in which a vegetarian diet was followed, group meditation and Sufi dancing were regular events, and there were both encounter groups and massage groups. The commune even had a resident guru who assisted the members along the spiritual path.

The people who lived in the commune ranged from naive students to middle-aged professionals (also naive possibly) and included a traditionally trained psychiatrist who practiced a curious blend of scientific and metaphysical medicine. In spite of the apparent diversity of the members of the group, they were all middle-class Americans who regularly chose to see both scientific and metaphysical healers. For them, the impersonalized and dehumanized aspects of contemporary medicine have made other forms of healing more attractive.

Health professionals in the United States believe there

are marked differences in the quality and character of rational medicine and so-called fringe medicine. Most traditional health care professionals do not recognize or give much credence to any alternative healing system. The adversary character of the relationship between scientific and metaphysical healing in this country causes many problems for the metaphysical healers and for the people who want their services. Let's take a close look at these difficulties; adequate and appropriate health care for our communities is at stake. Why are the various health belief systems unable to cooperate in an atmosphere of mutual respect and trust?

The detractors of alternative healing methods are vehement and direct about their objections. They say that metaphysical healing is essentially ineffective; that metaphysical healers are frequently irresponsible charlatans; that a patient's belief in an alternative healer often stands in the way of early medical detection of serious organic illness by an accredited physician; that there are irreconcilable conflicts between folk healing practices and rational medicine; and that belief in supernatural forces and paranormal events is not mentally healthy.

Most of the remainder of this chapter will be devoted to disagreement with this negative position, and to showing how cooperation between scientific and metaphysical healing will result in a mutual enrichment that will benefit the people they both serve.

First, of course, there would be economic benefits to both patients and scientific healers. There are many psychosomatic and psychiatric problems that can be dealt with by a folk healer. Many of the patients of the medical internist are actually suffering from emotional difficulties. This type of patient absorbs much of the physician's time, requires many fruitless laboratory tests, requests many changes in therapy, and experiences little relief—an obvious mismatch of patient and healer.

If physicians and folk healers were cooperating, dangers

of a misdiagnosis would be minimized. Metaphysical healers are often aware of their limitations and direct patients to physicians when appropriate. They would certainly do more of this if encouraged to do so. The reverse rarely occurs.

And there are other reasons for cooperation. Folk healers are frequently more integrated with the people of their community than are the scientific medical professionals; communication between the folk healer and the orthodox health care system would reduce some of the inundation and over-utilization that plague medicine today; scientific physicians are unable to respond to many inquiries from patients because they are over-trained or lack time.

There are both biological and emotional causes for illness. The causality can be very complex. Take the experience of a man we will call Steve, who had a vicious quarrel with his wife one day at breakfast. He left his house in a daze, stumbled on the porch steps, and tumbled into some shrubbery, badly scratching his hand. The hand soon became infected and Steve's family doctor gave him an injection of antibiotics. Steve had a violent allergic reaction. His condition became so critical he was hospitalized. As a child Steve had had a traumatic experience in a hospital, and his admission to his small private room now triggered bizarre behavior. He was moved to a high-security psychiatric ward. Can you imagine Steve's feelings as he lay nervously in bed looking at his infected hand and his grouchy wife? What was the cause of Steve's plight and what type of healer would you recommend? For an accurate diagnosis and effective therapy in such a case there must be understanding and manipulation of all factors. The folk healer deals more with the personal and social dynamics behind the illness while the scientific physician understands organic dysfunction best.

All of us have wondered why we can't have our body and mind treated simultaneously when we experience

36

some malady. Clearly the two are connected, and what we know about that connection will be explored in Chapter 5. The problem is that we do not yet know enough about the interdependence of mind and body. There is no single healer who has the skill and knowledge to provide a therapy intended for the whole person. Yet the basic characters of scientific healing and metaphysical healing should make them complementary, and in combination, capable of treating the whole person.

The fact is, however, that the concepts and beliefs underlying most metaphysical healing are unacceptable to the scientifically-minded and materialistically-oriented physician. The realities perceived by the two healers are so different. A doctor agreeing to the existence of spirits is as likely as a folk healer observing without repulsion a surgeon cutting into a human body. Because they have such different views of reality it is very difficult for the two types of healers to recognize that many treatment styles, techniques, and therapies are common to both ways of healing.

The most important argument for cooperation between scientific and metaphysical healers is that cooperation would increase the knowledge and capacity of both for healing. For example, digitalis, reserpine, cocaine, quinine, and psychedelic drugs—all revolutionary contributions to scientific medicine—were all first introduced as folk medicine. It seems scientific healers have short memories. So many folk healing procedures have been "discovered" by science and become a part of scientific theories, and yet there is continued attempted repression by health professionals of folk healing activities. The most important contributions of folk healing, surely, are yet to come. The body-mind connection is not well understood, and scientific medicine treats the body primarily. Until holistic medicine is actually being practiced, supportive interaction between the two styles will be more valuable than either style alone.

To reinforce this point, let's look at nine folk healing tools which are similar to those being used or considered for use in scientific healing: *ventilation, abreaction and catharsis, emotional and physical shock, conversion, persuasion and suggestion, group dynamics, psychodrama, dream interpretation,* and *music.*

A telephone call late at night and the strained voice of a friend saying, "I've just got to talk to you," is a form of *ventilation* we've all experienced. The opportunity to unburden oneself by talking about problems and sharing difficulties is known to be helpful at every level of human interaction. The value of ventilation is high when we are confessing objectionable facts to a tolerant and forgiving listener. If the confession is made to a group or to a person of authority, the ventilation has the most punch of all. Well-known examples are confessions in the Catholic Church and in the peyote ceremonies of North American Indians, and testifying at a Pentecostal church. Eskimos collectively confess their sins as part of a ritual in which their shaman, at the request of a sick person, goes symbolically to the bottom of the ocean to seek advice from the Mother of the Sea Beasts. The healing ceremony hinges on each participant confessing all wrongdoing and breaches of taboo, then repenting.

If a person experiences a traumatic event, it is not uncommon for him or her to bottle up the anxiety, shame, and mental anguish associated with the episode. This stored misery, unless released and dealt with, can have a harmful effect on the individual's functioning. In conventional psychotherapy, *abreaction* releases the repressed emotion, and spilling it all or *catharsis* brings release from tension and a sense of renewal.

Healing ceremonies often invoke abreaction and catharsis with massive emotional and physical energy discharges. Among the Shamburu pastoral nomads of northern Kenya a trance state with shaking and extreme physical agitation

38

is an acceptable way for unmarried men to deal with tension, danger, and frustration.

A dancing mania occurred at the time of the plagues of medieval Europe. In those difficult periods of misery and deprivation, masses of abused and underprivileged people were in some way inspired to dance wildly until they collapsed exhausted, temporarily at peace with the world.

The metaphysician thinks of abreaction as a way of counteracting spirit-possession. The catharsis is often simply a way of expressing unacceptable feelings. In Haiti there are few acceptable ways of being aggressive. If a Haitian is diagnosed as being possessed by *Limba,* one of the coarser Haitian voodoo gods, he or she can openly cavort in a drunken and greedy manner and enjoy whatever bizarre behavior is needed. In a culture in which there is no acceptable way to be greedy, gluttonous, or aggressive, this means of discharging negative energy is valuable. It is also in line with contemporary psychoanalytic ideas which hold that the only way to deal with highly negative feelings is to experience them by some means, and then healing can take place. There are countless psychological records that support the cleansing and simplifying effect of a dynamic discharge of feeling or of reliving the specific emotional content of a previous experience of one's life.

Emotional and physical shock have been used in many venerable healing methods. In ancient India mentally ill people were exposed to the attack of defanged cobras, to the charge of an elephant trained to stop at the last moment, or to fake arrest by the royal guard and sentencing to death. The intent was to invoke overwhelming fear and in this way to dispel the insanity.

Historically in Europe the mentally ill were treated by inducing hunger and using chains, beatings, torture, bloodletting, and forced laxatives. In England, Charles Darwin's grandfather, Erasmus Darwin (1731-1802), invented various swings and centrifuges in which the patient was rotated to the point of urinating, defecating, and losing consciousness. Not until tranquilizers appeared in the late 1950s was there a reduction in the use of a variety of shock treatments by European and American healers.

In Haiti, a voodoo ritual is used to rid epileptics of the evil spirits that are presumably causing their seizures. First the patient is purified by bathing; his clothes are burned and the ashes are mixed with indigo; then a deep cut is made in his arm and he is bled. A coating of the ash-indigo mixture is spread over his entire body except for the wound area.

The preparations are done by the *hungon* (the voodoo doctor) in a ritual of incredible intensity and emotion that culminates in the collapse of the patient. Now the patient is in a state of shock but still conscious, and the hungon plants in his mind suggestions intended to help the patient control his fits.

Another folk healing method which has been studied and acknowledged by Western medicine is *conversion*—a sudden and dramatic personality change. Religious conversion was considered the best remedy for alcoholism in the early 1900s, and through the Alcoholics Anonymous program, which essentially converts alcoholics, conversion remains the most effective form of treatment.

With conversion, there is a radical reversal of feelings, values, attitudes, and behavior of the converted person. Most often religious conversion is experienced by the individual who has been a heretic or an atheist. A person who was previously frivolous, promiscuous, and sexually uninhibited can be changed to lead a highly moral and ascetic life.

The interactions of people in large groups can provide fertile ground for conversion. Members of the audiences of a John Wesley or a Billy Sunday testify to "finding the path." The number of such testimonials is generally taken as a sign of the success of an evangelist.

Healing ceremonies frequently contain elements of *persuasion, suggestion,* and *hypnosis.* Early psychotherapists used these tools to treat a broad range of mental disorders. Perhaps the most unusual use of these techniques was by a Soviet psychiatrist in the early 1950s. His hysterical patients were made to wait in the hospital for several weeks until a difficult-to-obtain, rare, and expensive medicine was obtained. During the waiting period each patient was exposed to positive comments from the hospital staff regarding the value of the forthcoming treatment. Finally, the patient was moved to the operating room, where he overheard the doctors talking among themselves about the past successes of this treatment and the gratitude of cured patients. The patient was told that the drug would take exactly sixty seconds to work and that there would be only the one opportunity for treatment.

A mask was then placed over the patient's face and a dose of four drops of a harmless aromatic liquid was given. The result of the intensive suggestion and persuasion period was an impressive recovery rate for the psychiatrist's patients although some of his colleagues raised moral objections. The use of sugar pills, or placebos, has a fascinating history which we will review in Chapter 5.

Metaphysical healers often invoke in their patients special states of mind believed to be conducive to healing. In Haitian voodoo ceremonies the combination of music, dancing, and singing in the group setting invoke a hypnotic trance state. Especially the rhythm of the drum sets the mood of the ritual. There are endless examples of autohypnosis in religious experiences. Candle light, the cadence of speech, the chanting of prayers, and rhythmic body movements all influence the mood of the participants. In the extreme, there is evidence that persuasion and suggestion have been used to cause death. Voodoo cults claim to be able to cause psychological deaths, in which death is wished on, or suggested to, a victim by placing a hex on him or her. Such a death hex is usually used only on a person who is known to be inclined to hopelessness. Obviously, this is an example of the most negative use of suggestion.   41

Modern group psychotherapy and ancient healing ceremonies both use the power of *group dynamics.* Feelings of isolation, alienation, and morbid self-absorption are often reduced by interacting with other people in a supportive setting. In the trance dance of the African Kung bushmen, healing powers are believed to be transmitted by physical contact. The healing powers have to be reduced by passing through several people before being directed to the sick man. In this way, physical contact is maximized. It is a marvelously strengthening experience to learn in a psychotherapy group that you can be accepted by the group in spite of all your weaknesses, and to realize that others have similar problems. In both these cases the combined strength of the group actually heals.

In *psychodrama,* plays are spontaneously developed as the participants act out scenes and conflicts from their own lives. Because everyone, including the therapist, participates, this special technique allows the patient to see himself or herself through the eyes of other people. In this most unusual way the patient can see his own inner drives, emotions, and conflicts. In a related technique for metaphysical healing, a shaman acts out a life or death struggle between his own spirit and the evil spirit causing the individual's sickness.

Another situation, identified as spirit possession, involved a young woman who had been depressed for several months. She was induced into a trance by a folk healer. The woman went back to her childhood and enacted not only her own role but that of her mother. The healer's continuous suggestions and involvement isolated a conflict and the guilt related to it. When the woman left the trance state she was questioned by the healer. The childhood-related guilt seemed to have dissipated and the depression lifted.

Dream interpretation was used by metaphysical healers long before it was discovered by psychology and psychiatry. In the Greco-Roman period, priests of the temples of

Asklepious used dream oracles to divine the nature of an illness and to foretell the future.

Consider the culture of the Senoi, who live on the central mountain range of Malaya. Much of their life is extremely primitive—no irrigation or fertilization of land and no domestic animals. Food is supplied primarily from hunting and from gathering jungle products. In startling contrast, their emotional education and interpersonal relations are perhaps the most highly developed that humans have been able to attain. Violent crime is unknown among them. There is no use of alcohol or any other drug. Mental illness does not appear to exist for the Senoi. Their families, their economy, and their healing system operate well on the principles of contract, agreement, and consensus.

The culture of the Senoi revolves around dreams and psychodrama. A child, as soon as he or she is able, shares his dreams with members of his family. They all listen carefully, and regardless of the nature of the dream, support the idea that all dream characters are potentially good. The children are instructed to approach all the friendly dream images with appreciation and to ask them for interesting and useful contributions for their friends and family. Eventually every child finds a dream character who is his or her permanent guide and advisor.

All the Senoi, including the children, participate in ceremonial dances involving a group trance. Dream characters are invited to visit the dreamer during the dance. A bargain is made in which the dream character agrees to possess the dancer if some condition is satisfied. Typical conditions include learning a dance or song, creating a design, or following some dietetic restriction.

At the climax of the dance, the young dancers fall writhing to the ground as if seized by a fit. Boys, encouraged by the old men, go deep into the violent stage of the trance. Assuming the fetal position, they jabber incoherently while the men talk to them, massage them, and slap them with sacred leaves. Apparently by choice, Senoi girls

43

do not usually seek this stage of possession in the ceremony. As the peak of the fit passes, the boys become coherent and describe and share their experiences with other members of the community.

The trance dance and its preparations occupy a great deal of the time of the Senoi. Their days are spent making perishable dance costumes, gathering sacred plants, collecting flowers and resins for the dream characters, rehearsing songs and dances, conducting healing ceremonies, carrying out expeditions and courtships required by the dream companions and attending daily meetings for interpretation of dreams. Is it any wonder that their technological development is so limited? The mini culture of the Senoi is a fascinating antithesis of our technological culture.

The years that the Senoi child spends in these activities result in a well-integrated adult in whom catharsis is easily induced. The dreaming practices of the children encourage experimentation with the inner world. The child comes to terms with his or her inner world by doing whatever he or she dreams about, whether it be writing a poem or building some gadget. The poem is then read to the community (or the gadget is tested) and exposed to criticism. The actual consummation of all dream activities is encouraged.

Recent scientific studies have shown that certain dreams precede the onset of particular organic diseases at a stage where modern laboratory testing could not reliably detect the diseases. Heeding our dreams may lead to new skills for early diagnosis.

Another tool of metaphysical healing that is making an impact on scientific therapy is *music*. In all times and all cultures music has accompanied the important events of people's lives. Music was an important part of healing ceremonies in the Greek temples of Askleois. In Saturn's temple on the Nile riverboat cruises with music and dancing were used to treat the mentally ill.

In our times the role of music in Navajo healing ceremonies is especially important. Their curing rites are actually called chants or sings. More than fifty Navajo healing rituals are dedicated to their belief that evil can be overcome and order restored through the proper use of ceremonies. The Navajos do not require confession or self-examination to get well. Their healing chants overcome the supernatural. The complexity of their personal healing ritual has been compared to the task of memorizing a Wagnerian opera, including the orchestral score, all vocal parts, setting details, stage movements, and costume requirements. The Navajos believe that a person's body cannot be treated without treating the soul, and vice versa. The patient is viewed as a total person—body, attitudes, and responsibilities. The line between physical and mental illness is blurred. The idea of sickness encompasses far more than broken bones, cuts, burns, and the like.

Music therapists are now among the specialists of modern Western psychiatry. Music is an integral part of such innovations in psychotherapy as guided fantasy, bioenergetics, encounter groups, and marathons. Music plays an important role in psychedelic therapy.

There you have it: A smorgasbord of nine connections between metaphysical healing and modern scientific medicine. The list of old, new, and developing connections between metaphysical healing and scientific healing is essentially endless. The two are not separate and unrelated areas of human endeavor.

The major difference between the two spheres of healing, metaphysical and scientific, is in the perception of reality by their healers and patients, and, springing from this, their ways of perceiving illness and getting well. In Chapter 2, the African and American perceived the world very differently from one another. History teaches us that people see the world in a variety of ways. Viewpoints range between two distant extremes. One view of the world is founded on these principles: Matter is real and solid; we learn about the world only through our senses; causes must precede effects; objects separated by space are different objects. Complete belief in and acceptance of these basic principles confines the nature of our experience. We are described as being rational. The act of bending a piece of metal merely by thinking of it is inconceivable. The scientific healer is in this rational camp.

At the other extreme of reality is a set of mystical principles: There is a better way of learning about the world than through the senses; there is a basic unity of all things; there is no reality in time; all evil is mere appearance. Though it over-simplifies, we might think of the two viewpoints as those of the intellectual observer and the emotional perceiver.

I have two friends who exemplify these extremes of reality. Joan is extremely bright but absolutely non-intellectual (not anti-intellectual). She operates directly on emotional energy and other kinds of energy best described as psychic and mystic. She is instinctively accepting of everything occult. Her life is filled at times with bizarre experiences, but she has a kind of insulation from any negative effects. She has told me that when something I would call evil or cruel is happening to her, it is as though her essence can climb out of her skin, stand aside, and wait until her body can be recovered again.

All the diverse parts of Joan's life are tied together. At the market she may select vegetables by closing her eyes and sensing the energy from the zucchini she wants. Joan follows up an advertisement on the market bulletin board because the name on the advertisement triggers memories of a person who appeared in a dream she had the previous night.

Bruce, on the other hand, is a rational, organized, intellectual man. The *whys* of everything are important to him. He lives by inference. When I meet him I can almost hear the whirr as he mentally gathers information and evidence that will guide his actions in the next moment. When Bruce has to come to a decision he makes a list of all the alternatives open to him, then speculates on what would happen to him if he made a particular choice. When his analysis is complete he chooses the option that offers the most reward to him.

It has been proposed by some researchers and philosophers who have tried to reconcile various views of reality that the physical objects of our life are set in the three dimensions of reality that are accessible to our consciousness in a fourth dimension of time. Total reality, however, would include up to six other dimensions that we cannot detect with our usual senses. Psychic phenomena, which fall within the six other dimensions, are perceived by only a few people. All of this is only an idea, but it seems clear that in time scientific principles will be introduced into mysticism and mystical notions into science. When this happens psychology (scientific) and parapsychology (metaphysical) will be reconciled. The tie between scientific and metaphysical healing will become formal. Cooperation between our metaphysical healers and our health professionals will be a reality.

We have been discussing ways to heal, but a critical point has so far been omitted. None of the many healers referred to in this book *actually heal.* They provide suitable conditions and *assist the body in healing itself.*

If you ask healers how they heal, some answers might be:

"I don't heal, the Holy Spirit heals through me."

"I just make it possible for your natural healing energies to flow."

"I drive away the demons who are making you sick."

"I change your environment so you will get well."

"I put things back in order, then I help your body heal itself."

There are as many answers as there are types of healers. The last answer given above might have come from an honest and enlightened physician. Physicians study the body while it heals itself. No other healer is as interested in

47

the scientific details of healing as the doctor, but of course that is his or her background, training, and inclination.

The physician works from a scientific model of the process of the body healing itself. Take the example of a broken leg. The doctor has an X ray taken and, based on that special look inside the leg, he manipulates the bones until they are in proper alignment. He applies a plaster cast to maintain the alignment and his work is done.

The physician hasn't healed the broken bone—he has just created a set of conditions enabling the body to proceed with healing the fracture. Here is how the doctor visualizes what the body does: At the bone break there is some bleeding from the marrow cavity of the bone and from the torn blood vessels in the fat and muscle around the bone. The blood begins to clot at the break, forming a mixture of agents including a protein. The area of the break is completely cleaned of debris and crushed tissue by special cells that have migrated in the blood stream to the damaged area. Other bone-building cells begin to repair the bone in a way that is not understood. Somehow calcium is supplied from the blood stream to the mixture of agents in the clotted blood at the break. In six to eight weeks this mixture turns into bone and the leg is solidly mended.

Most other healers would insist that by their procedures, their rituals, or sheerly by charisma, patients are stimulated to heal more rapidly than they otherwise might. Doctors have observed the variation in healing rates among their patients, and probably would not disagree with these healers' claims. A famous British surgeon always insisted that his personality contributed much more to healing than did his scalpel.

Most of us grew up under the care of a traditional physician, so we will take a careful look at him or her in the next chapter, then return to the issue of charismatic stimulation of healing in Chapter 5.

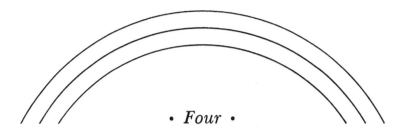

Scientific Medicine

The American doctor is in deep trouble. In the midst of what has been called "the Golden Age of Medicine," our modern scientific healers must brace themselves for a major wave of reformation.

In fairness, given our national health problems and the expectations of our society—a house of cards that we have constructed from our faith in science and technology—any doctor who could meet all our needs would have to be a superbeing. He or she would have to be rich in compassion, humanism, wisdom, logic, analytical ability, technical expertise, scholarship, morality, honesty, political acumen, originality, legal knowledge, and journalistic and oratorical skill, with a suitable disposition, a sense of history, and extraordinary mental and physical endurance. A mountain of material has been written about what happens when a physician fails to possess one or more of these attributes. As a culture we stand by and express amazement when a scientific house of cards is revealed as weak and about to tumble down.

We need not pull yet another card from that mythic structure. The practical intention of this book is to examine the real record of the American doctor as a healer and to consider why an increasing numer of Americans have lost faith and are seeking metaphysical healers.

A much publicized condition that probably influences many of our citizens to seek alternative healing is our rank with respect to health among the other developed nations of the world. We rank twenty-fifth in lifespan, fourteenth in both infant and mother survival in childbirth, and eighth in the ratio of doctors to patients. Yet we spend more money per capita on health care than any other nation of the world. To go on with the litany of unhappy statistics, at least five thousand American communities don't have a doctor, some twenty million Americans receive little or no health care, and more than six million persons suffer from severe or incurable handicaps.

To read of marvelous medical advances on one page of a newspaper and then to be told of health privation on another page leads us to the horrid suspicion that all is not well. A success with a new kind of heart valve is counterbalanced by an article about the effects of malnutrition on children living in isolated mountain communities. The more our health industry grows, and the larger the demands made on it, the less health we find.

Disease appears to be a Hydra-headed monster. When we have conquered one disease, others even more difficult to control appear in its place. Most infectious fevers have been eliminated only to be replaced by diseases that attack the central nervous system.

The number of deaths at birth has been lowered substantially, but a growing number of middle-aged people are struck down in the prime of life by a heart attack or stroke. One person in seven has some form of rheumatism or arthritis. We win the war against tuberculosis only to be confronted with an increase in the incidence of cancer, especially cancer of the lung. We master the acute microbic diseases only to be beaten by new and unmanageable virus infections. Psychotherapies and therapists proliferate, and Americans, more than ever before, have immersed themselves in an orgy of mental analysis with uncertain results. Never have we known so much about disease and pathological conditions and so little about health and wholeness.

We now see the patient's loss of confidence in the physician reflected in the rapid increase in malpractice charges. In 1968 one in eight doctors were sued for malpractice; in 1974 it was one in four. In the past decade the average malpractice claim grew from $6,000 to $23,400. Juries are granting many more awards in the million-dollar category.

Then there are the problems of the patients who simply don't go to physicians any more. Some of these people will seek and find other kinds of healers, but many other individuals who turn away from doctors do without any medical services.

Many points of view about scientific healing are available, but there is one that is never sought and is rarely offered: What does the metaphysician think of the scientific physician?

A story is told of a research team of African metaphysicians that was funded by the United Nations to study doctors and medicine in the United States. The head of the team, Dr. Baba, a witch doctor from the jungles of West Africa, was to supervise the preparation of a report intended to acquaint the various associations of tribal healers in their respective countries with American medicine.

It was Dr. Baba's first trip away from his native jungle village, and his team had been visiting health facilities in New York City less than a week when the study was abruptly terminated. In a most mysterious fashion funding was cut off and the members of the team were flown back to their countries before any interviews could take place. Except for the diligent efforts of a cub reporter, nothing would have been known here of Dr. Baba's reaction to healing in this country. The young journalist intercepted the contents of a wastebasket from Dr. Baba's hotel room and recovered crumpled notes written by the famous healer. These scraps of writing were pieced together to form the following paragraphs in Dr. Baba's words:

In New York all sick people must leave their village and go to the house of a medicine man just to get a naming-of-sickness. After a long wait a sick man has learned much about other sickness from sick people who wait with him.

The medicine man looks inside the body with special medicine that damages the body. He cannot see the spirits of dead ancestors or the colored light around the head made by a sick man's spirit.

I saw spirits rolling on the floor and having a good laugh when the medicine man tried to scare spirit with black ropes in the ears to look like snakes and a large, round shiny eye on the forehead.

American medicine men still do the cutting medicine which we gave up many centuries ago. Only the sick man's will to live and the spirits of his ancestors allow him to survive this barbarism and mutilation. Population is controlled in my country by famine and in the United States by cutting medicine.

Poisoning medicine has nearly replaced roots-and-flowers medicine of the past. Now entire villages are supported by gold they receive for making poisoning medicine. Poisoning medicine is used to drive the sick man's spirit out when body parts are going to be cut off. Sometimes a sick man doesn't have enough ancestors to save him from both the poison and the cutting.

Must remember to send copies of our journals on roots-and-flower medicines because the poisons do more harm to the body than the sickness does.

Equipment is very poor. Saw spirits falling asleep with boredom because of no imagination with masks and costumes. Not one rattle did I see.

The worst thing I saw was the epidemic of gold sickness—especially the medicine men. Dreams of gold sap their energy for healing. So many Americans make themselves sick by chasing dreams of gold. We know about gold sickness and must teach American medicine men special prayers which cure the gold sickness.

In the guarded houses for people with crazy sickness I saw such terrible things. Poisoning, cutting, and machines which make a sick man tremble like a leaf in a hurricane. But mostly so much talking. U.S. medicine does not even know how to start treatment of people

52

with evil spirits controlling their minds. They do not know the proper ceremonies.

Some of the other sorcerers, shamans, and witch doctors want to offer foreign aid to the Americans. We will send gold which we do not need and this will be given to the American medicine men if they will stop their primitive and superstitious practices.

In exchange the United States will send us their crazy people. The possessed among them will be exorcised and returned home in a few days. Those with the spirit vision will be kept and trained in our medical ways: modern demonology, aura reading, use of natural substances, energy balancing with needles, mask-making and such.

Our gift of these modern medical ways will cement our friendship to America as no other gift will. If only I can survive the food available here, I am going to support this proposal when I return to my village.

This is only a story and it may be a fantasy to think of such cooperation between scientific and metaphysical healers, but Dr. Baba's proposal contains a lot of common sense.

Let's take a close look at allopathy, which is the basis of the healing techniques of the traditional physician. Allopathic methods were developed in Europe after the Renaissance as healers looked for a new approach to convincing patients that something active and successful was being done on their behalf. Prayers and incantations were no longer effective. These new methods were based on a doctrine of contraries derived from the teachings of a medical sect which existed in Asia Minor in the first century B.C. The principle of allopathy is straightforward: any deviation from the body's normal functioning is controlled by applying a counteracting procedure. People with chills are warmed and those with fevers are cooled.

In the fifteenth century illness was thought to be related to the presence in the body of toxic and foreign materials, so techniques focused on their elimination. Every imaginable method was employed to purge the body of poisons. Irritants and drugs were used as well as barbaric bleedings, cuppings, enemas, and the like.

The healing viewpoint at that time emphasized the allopathic notion and purging. There was no scientific explanation for this viewpoint. Healing was based on theories handed down from the past, and was characterized by a whirlwind of contrary treatments. Allopathic medication was harsh, and few doctors dared to recommend rest and quiet for their patients. To leave patient recovery to the natural life force would have been admission that medicine had no specific treatments to offer.

It is likely that these cruel and essentially powerless allopathic medications, which continued on into the late nineteenth century, would have faded away, leaving only an unpleasant taste in the mouth of humanity, except for a historical coincidence. A rival medical theory, homeopathy, was founded by Samuel Hahnemann, a German physician, in 1796 and quickly became popular and apparently successful in healing. Homeopathy's central principle is that treatments should be given that cause symptoms like those of the illness—let likes be treated by likes. I will discuss homeopathy in detail later; the point here is that homeopathic physicians promoted an approach to illness that was the reverse of allopathy.

A fierce battle soon developed between the two rival, unsubstantiated healing theories—one that would last 100 years. Then the French chemist Louis Pasteur discovered germs. In a flash, divine vengeance, cosmic forces, witchcraft, emanations, and evil spirits gave way to tiny wiggling organisms as the causes of illness.

Never before had any concrete cause for illness been known. Allopaths immediately jumped on the bandwagon, claiming that they had been saying all along that illness was caused by outside agents, even if they hadn't known what the agents were. Now allopathic treatments could be aimed at combating germs. Use of the proper drugs would eliminate germs and cure the accompanying illness.

By this quirk of historical timing, order came out of medical chaos just before the dawn of the twentieth century. All sorts of different healers had at last found a cohesive, binding force. Homeopathy faded and allopathy flourished. Allopathic medication became one of three foundation stones of modern medicine, the others being surgery and immunization. *Medicine* has become the generic term for *allopathic medicine* to such a degree that it is a rare American who has ever heard the word *allopathy*. Both allopathic and homeopathic pharmacies still exist in Europe, however, and the American tourist who chooses the wrong one is in for a surprise.

The popularity of the allopathic approach to medicine is especially interesting and ironic in the light of Louis Pasteur's deathbed conclusion. Almost his last words were to the effect that the microbe mattered less than the mental and physical ground on which it was let loose, a sentiment that supports the technique of immunization, clearly an integral element of traditional medicine in the 1970s. Yet innoculation is a *homeopathic* idea. Weak germs of a particular disease are injected into humans, who then build up antibodies and thus acquire immunity from the real germs that may strike later on. The procedure improves the body before the onslaught of disease rather than waiting to attack the germs once disease has invaded the body.

Nevertheless, for the next fifty years the success of allopathic medicine made homeopathy and all other forms of healing unpopular. Only the old-fashioned, ignorant, and superstitious used other systems of medicine, but no attempt was made to suppress alternative healers in this period as long as they didn't pretend to be qualified physicians. Many of the new germ-slaying allopathic drugs worked with happy results. Diseases that had haunted mankind for centuries were conquered or rendered insignificant. Causality is difficult to determine, however. During this same period standards of living dramatically improved as did all social services.

By the mid-twentieth century, the weaknesses of the allopathic method were becoming starkly apparent to any medical critic or professional who would look.

Sulfa drugs and antibiotics had contributed spectacularly to banishing a number of specific diseases, but disease was as widespread as ever. All health services were jammed. But, here again, causality is difficult to determine. Population had increased, due partly to the success of drugs, and the people who were now living longer were experiencing the strokes, rheumatism, and cancer of advanced years. A higher standard of living and employment meant more people were demanding to be treated for disorders that previously would have been tolerated in the imposed silence of poverty. While plagues and many other maladies had been virtually eliminated by the mid-twentieth century, an explosion of disorders of the respiratory system, of the circulation, of digestion, of the body's cells and tissues, and especially of neuroses, was occurring.

In order to understand the functioning of the modern physicians, who are molded in the allopathic tradition, let's briefly review their training. First there is graduation from medical school, where the indoctrination is based on a healing model that reflects variations of the allopathic theme. After completing a one- or two-year internship and passing a state licensing examination, doctors can, in theory, practice any kind of medicine they choose—from prescribing medication for a cold to performing brain surgery.

Once a state licenses physicians it virtually washes its hands of them. Unless physicians break laws, become addicted to narcotics, or attract attention in some extremely bizarre way, all they have to do is pay an annual license fee and the state leaves them alone. The explosion in medical information generally makes the fledging doctor obsolete in six or seven years, but no re-examination is required.

In an effort to make it possible for a doctor to be particularly competent in some field, twenty-two medical specialties have evolved, ranging from anesthesiology to urology. To become a specialist a physician must serve a residency training period in a hospital and then pass a stiff examination given by a board composed of doctors in that field. The residencies take two to four years to complete, and some stalwart souls go beyond that to sub-specialties such as the treatment of heart disease or gastro-intestinal problems.

Board certification doesn't guarantee a specialist's competence but is a reasonable indicator of competence. Under state laws, however, any doctor can claim to be a specialist without board certification and patients are rarely the wiser. Half the specialists in internal medicine are not certified—nor are 45 per cent of the specialists in obstetric-gynecology, nearly half of the psychiatrists and anesthesiologists, 30 per cent of the general surgeons, and 20 per cent of the pediatricians. The state doesn't care about all this, but it may mean everything to the patient suffering from the type of organic dysfunction in which the allopathic physician excells.

Studies show that when early cancer of the cervix is operated on by qualified board-certified gynecologists, there is an 80 per cent cure rate. When the operation is performed by doctors without these qualifications, the rate of cure is only 50 per cent.

Neither physicians nor medical societies have done much to promote quality control. Patients who seek the special skills of the scientific healer are thrown on their own to judge the treatment they have received. It's a job the typical, passive patient can't do. In a survey taken in a New York hospital, 75 per cent of the patients who had received the worst medical care, according to professional evaluation, thought they had actually received the best.

The highly scientific educational process of the doctor steers him or her toward the job of technologist and away from the role of comforter of the sick; yet most patients

57

need a healer who will take a personal interest in them while the body does its own natural healing.

After diagnosis, the two main tools of the scientific doctor are drugs and surgery. Lack of knowledge and sophistication in the use of drugs has been cited as the greatest deficiency of the average physician today. One report identified medical schools in which only a single course in drugs and their uses was offered.

The average hospital patient receives no fewer than nine different drugs during his or her stay. The estimated thirty thousand hospital patients who die annually from drug reactions receive only a tiny fraction of the publicity given to the fifty thousand deaths on our highways each year. A 1975 survey taken in New York showed that one child in five had received antibiotics for viral infection even though it has been shown that antibiotics are of no help in fighting viruses.

As the allopathic physician's arsenal of drugs has increased, side effects or allergies to the drugs have also increased. By the 1960s, *iatrogenic illness,* as disorders caused by medical treatment came to be called, had taken its place as one of the most widespread of mankind's medical difficulties. The documentation for the undesirable effects of drugs is substantial. As one doctor put it, "Bark tea and ground-up goats' testicles didn't do much of anything, but they didn't make the patient sicker either."

The new drugs accomplish what they are supposed to—they kill bacteria, prevent infection, and suppress inflamation—but the very strength that allows them to do these tasks disturbs the body organism in many ways. It's literally a chemist's nightmare. There are first, second, third, and so on side effects both from the illness and the drugs, and all of these unpredictable results interact. I'm not being particularly facetious to suggest yet another specialty that would be in immediate demand—Doctor of Iatrogenic Medicine.

58

The incredible aspect of this subject is that by using the scientific approach doctors surely must have seen whether a drug worked and should have discarded it if it did not give positive results. Why it does not always work this way is worth exploring further.

Allopathic drugs have been evolving for centuries, and long ago doctors realized that the usefulness of a drug could not simply be determined by trying it on a group of patients. Of course, if such a test killed all the patients, the drug was discarded. But if the patients all recovered the doctors could only speculate as to which caused the cure, the drug or the natural life force. The speedy recovery of an essentially healthy child who is limp with a 104° fever at two in the morning, but wakes up for breakfast with energy, vitality, and a big appetite could be mistakenly attributed to a drug's effect.

Long ago doctors recognized that the value of a drug was deeply connected to the patient's belief in it. Often suggestibility would cause colored water to have the impact of a potent drug, but not for everyone. Doctors and quacks have both taken advantage of this phenomenon, calling it "the placebo effect," from the Latin, "I will please." The placebo has become a staple of controlled drug evaluation. In trying to determine the value of a drug, half the patients in a test group are given the drug and the other half a placebo.

This scientific approach seems rational, but another amazing effect has emerged. Some new drugs that have come through controlled studies with flying colors seem to lose their potent effects as time goes on. It has long been clear that the success of a drug, or any therapeutic treatment for that matter, depends not only on the patient's attitude, but also on the doctor's. If the doctor really believes in it, it works.

Cortisone is a classic example of a drug whose initial promise was not realized, and with cortisone yet another drug evaluation difficulty appeared. The purpose of cortisone was to eliminate inflammatory changes in tissues. Initially very successful in treating arthritis, it seemed reasonable to use it anywhere in the body that inflammation occurred. Ultimately the hormonal balance of the body was upset by cortisone and long-term secondary effects appeared: fatness and floridity, exhaustion of the adrenal glands, susceptibility to infection, peptic ulcers, and delayed healing of wounds, to name a few.

I want to emphasize that assessing the effects of drugs is very difficult. Different persons react differently to the same drug, side effects often take a long time to develop, and patient and doctor attitudes affect response to the drug.

The double-blind test was designed to eliminate the doctor's influence. In such a test neither the doctor, not the patient, nor anybody else in the hospital knows which patients are getting the new drug and which are getting the placebo. In cases like "the Pill," testing—and controversy about side effects—may go on for years. Testing drugs on animals doesn't help because animals and humans don't react in the same ways. As to the ethics and limits of testing drugs on humans, no one knows the answers. In spite of their inauspicious beginnings and checkered history, drugs increase in number each year. Drugs do have value, but they cannot be used mindlessly.

People find it hard to turn away from drugs that clear up distressing problems or allow them to sleep. Although a placebo effect may actually be at work, relief of some degree is often obtained. We are part of a culture with a low threshold for discomfort.

I have reviewed the use of drugs in traditional medicine at a time when there is escalating concern about iatrogenic illness. The charges are coming not only from sources hostile to allopathy. Orthodox medical journals frequently report research results that literally discredit the system that gives physicians their clinical creed.

60

As the controversies wear on, we would do well to bear in mind that traditional medical practitioners, through a combination of historical chance and confusion over causality as well as ends and means, decided long ago to make war on disease with chemical weapons. Over a period of some eighty years, our healers have turned us into test tubes.

An alternative is to fight disease with biological weapons. Germs and other minute pests are part of the evolutionary process and obey the law of survival of the fittest. The possibility of introducing their natural enemies to control them has not been given serious thought. Nor has there been support in this country for finding ways of making our bodies inhospitable to the invaders.

Consider the parallel to insecticides. A chemical attack was made on insect pests in the 1940s. Success was generally spotty, the balance of nature was disturbed, and usually the pests returned in a few years—resistant to the poisons that had previously killed them. As this is written, the trend is to return to biological control of insect pests.

Another speculation about allopathic medication is almost terrifying. There is impressive evidence that many persons fall ill in order to retreat from the excessive strain induced by our modern technological civilization. At these times their life force is protecting them from situations that are too much for them. Except for averting a physical catastrophe, using drugs does not assist the life force but opposes it. Some researchers believe that the battle that occurs between natural life forces and medication causes damaging side effects. No one knows for sure.

The public has been conditioned to expect miracles from allopathic drugs. Yet the triumphs over the pests which could be seen under the microscope have not been extended to degenerative disorders such as cancer and rheumatism. Unrealized high expectations in the patient-doctor relationship and growing malpractice charges are among the unpleasant results of patient disappointment.

The doctor's use of his other major tool, the scalpel, also receives increasing criticism. The major intention of surgery is to repair the damage of disease. The value of surgery in correcting acute conditions is unsurpassed from the viewpoint of scientific medicine. There is overwhelming evidence, however, that surgery is frequently used needlessly. For example, if we compare the surgical experience of the average American today to that of the average Briton we find that Britons undergo in their lifetimes only half as many operations as Americans. The typical British patient receives health services with a strong preventive emphasis. Surgery is the last option.

If the body has been poorly treated, or if the organism has malfunctioned so that a catastrophic organic failure is looming or has occurred, the surgeon appears. He is a court of last resort. There is nothing preventive about him; he deals in the here and now. He is concerned with specific matters like gallstones and tumors, and there is never any question about the laying on of hands. The surgeon is concerned with organic mutations and dysfunctions; and within the traditional allopathic model, the major criticism of the surgeon is that he or she performs too much unwarranted surgery.

Again, much has been written about needless surgery, but it is of more concern to me that surgery is a violation and mutilation of the body. The question always is whether the surgery may do more damage than the dysfunction it is intended to correct. There is no simple answer.

At one time—up to the 1950s—surgery was used to deal with stress symptoms. Costly, laborious, and dangerous brain surgery was performed on many thousands of mentally ill patients, only to have it discovered many years later that these procedures were of dubious value.

The place of surgery in orthodox medicine today is not

enviable. Desperate attempts to use the scientific approach take the form of endless experiments to determine whether one drug is better than another. Rarely is there consideration of an alternative to drug therapy unless it is surgery. The medical profession's fear of the unorthodox perpetuates the use of surgery in an unnatural way.

The trial and error approach to developing many of the techniques used in scientific healing is helpful only if doctors are aware of the results. Many doctors continued for fifteen years to prescribe a synthetic estrogen to prevent miscarriage despite six well-documented studies that showed the drug to be ineffective. Many doctors still recommend bed rest for persons with infectious hepatitis and people with ulcers still buckle down to bland diets, even though both procedures have been shown to be ineffective.

Physicians also exhibit a disturbing lack of knowledge of nutrition. Nutrition is a slippery subject about which too little is known, and even experts disagree. In an area where it is admittedly difficult to be knowledgable, the typical physician nevertheless seems singularly and oddly out of touch, and this especially angers patients today. On the other hand, the occasional nutrition maverick among doctors usually has little impact, expecially in the face of ethnic eating styles. Henry Bieler, however, has made some headway with his best selling book *Food Is Your Best Medicine.* In his notes to the reader he says:

As a practicing physician for over fifty years, I have reached three basic conclusions as to the cause and care of disease. This book is about those conclusions.

The first is that the primary cause of disease is not germs. Rather, I believe that disease is caused by a toxemia which results in cellular impairment and breakdown, thus paving the way for the multiplication and onslaught of germs.

The second conclusion is that in almost all cases the use of drugs in treating patients is harmful. Drugs often cause serious side effects, and sometimes even create new diseases. . . .

My third conclusion is that disease can be cured through the proper use of correct foods.

As an interesting aside, when queried by a patient as to whether his diet for her would be effective if prescribed by *any* doctor, Dr. Bieler, a believer in a healer's unique charismatic stimulation, replied negatively.

I have discussed some surface aspects of modern medicine's research, experimentation, and discovery, which are conducted in the name of improving health care. Sometimes these activities create shiny modern laboratories in hospitals where rain leaks in on the patients and some wards do not have adequate bathing facilities. Through this complex setting walks the physician, who is confronted by a patient's expectation that his or her every previous indulgence and excess can be remedied in a single medical visit. Is it any wonder that I have said the physician in this culture must be a superbeing?

Is the medical profession trying to extricate itself from the deficiencies of the allopathic method? Not really. There is too much professional ego wrapped up in the status quo. Most professions are protective associations and as such are highly resistant to change.

The nature of healing interaction seems to be that whatever the time or place, most of the population and the medical profession accept that the treatments in fashion are effective. It is also perennially believed that treatments are better than they used to be, but not as good as they will be. Medical disillusionments are a strange breed of cat. Instead of breeding scepticism, they only nourish fresh illusions, which are a complex form of the patient giving up his personal power.

Summing up to this point, the first half of the twentieth century was the heyday of allopathic medication. A mood of public acceptance prevailed which has been disintegrating only in the last decade. Generations of doctors have grown up regarding allopathy as the only orthodox medicine. Some attention is paid to preventive medicine in the same spirit as that of the uncultured person who occasionally attends the opera because he or she feels all the better for it for days after. There is little doubt, however, that curative medicine continues to be king of the mountain, and its weapons remain drugs and surgery.

The education of a traditional healer in our culture emphasizes the memorization of a mountain of technical and scientific material. There is little chance for humanistic broadening or even medical exploration in the training of a doctor. The learn-by-doing medical journeyman work takes precedence.

The focus on science in a doctor's training has been at the expense of developing therapeutic skills. As a result, the critical, irreplaceable therapeutic skill of a doctor with a patient hardly counts any more when determining the merit of a doctor. Many doctors find it easier to order a series of laboratory tests when making a diagnosis than to rely on their own senses.

We have all seen the laboratories. Rows of test tubes and chromium plated machines. Dark rooms and devices, both tiny and massive. Lead vests and scary needles. And many of us take it for granted that somewhere within all this mysterious machinery lies the truth about what is really wrong with us. Science strikes again!

Further softening of the certainty about science is necessary. Let's take a look at the *electroencephalogram*—the gadget that records brain waves. This fascinating-looking device is touted as a necessity for accurate diagnosis of a brain lesion, but a little reading in medical literature will dissuade many of that necessity. Fifteen to 20 per cent of all patients with clinically established convulsive disorders never have an abnormal electroencephalogram reading; the same percentage of the general population with no history of convulsive disorders gives abnormal readings.

What about our old friend, the X ray? If something's there, a picture will not lie. Don't be so sure. Medical surveys have shown that as many as 24 per cent of radiologists differed with each other in their interpretations of the same X ray films, even in cases of extensive disease. An even more unsettling statistic is that 31 per cent of radiologists disagreed with *themselves* when reading the same films at a later time.

Almost all of us have seen or heard of the *electrocardiogram,* which traces the beating of a heart. In one study, doctors changed their interpretations of the wiggly lines of the electrocardiogram 20 per cent of the time on rereading them later. Other studies have shown that electrocardiogram readings change enormously depending on the time of day, activity, digestive function, and personal characteristics. Identification of heart trouble amid all of this variation requires very careful interpretation and would hardly be called precise.

The laboratory technician and his procedures don't fare much better under scrutiny. When a red blood cell count was done by a number of technicians in one study, the technicians showed an error range from 16 to 28 per cent from the true value. When an electronic cell counter is used, the error is still at least 16 per cent. Such a magnitude of error could mask the presence of types of anemia. All laboratory results must be interpreted with extreme care. They can supplement, not replace, the senses and brains of the healer.

Most physicians support the notion that good medicine consists of rest, nursing, diet, and the use of drugs when required. This formula, when interpreted in the allopathic theme, is not as simple as it seems.

The main flaws in orthodox medicine are: assumption of effectiveness of theoretical therapies; assumption of validity for erroneous or unproven cause and effect relationships; failure to look at the patient as a whole; and overvaluation of technology.

The history of medicine has included trephining skulls to release the confined demon that was causing insanity; starvation to remove the basis of fever; resting patients for months or even years to improve the state of their hearts, livers, or brains; putting the wretched victims of ankylosing spendylitis on plaster beds for a year or two to reduce the inflammation; keeping patients in bed for weeks after an operation; and anteverting uteruses to cure backache. Some of these useless and sometimes harmful methods were used thousands of years ago; others, such as anteversion operations, were first used in this century.

Each of these remedies was developed because some unsubstantiated theory of the particular period argued that the remedy *must* be effective. When the remedy was used, it was easy to deduce that it *had* been effective since many patients improved or recovered.

Medicine today asks for evidence, not theory, to determine whether a remedy is valuable. We have seen how obtaining evidence of the value of drugs is incredibly difficult. Many general medical procedures still persist from earlier times in spite of the lack of evidence validating the procedures. Examples are: placing shock patients in a bed raised at the foot on blocks; advising bland foods for peptic ulcer patients; and ordering a fat-free diet for patients with infectious hepatitis.

In attempting to establish the causes of disease scientific medicine frequently makes errors of attribution. Symptoms are attributed to a pathological process that doesn't exist or is irrelevant to the patient's illness. I could fill pages with examples, but one intriguing case is enough. Symptoms were incorrectly supposed to be related to two types of gastritis in the 1930s, though gastritis had hardly existed in the 1920s. The invention of the flexible gastroscope apparently made gastritis popular for a few years and then it disappeared again.

67

Many patients who are wrongly diagnosed in this way have physical symptoms with an emotional basis. Lower back pain is an example of a difficulty that cannot rightly be attributed either to organic disease or to psychological disorder.

Scientific healers tend to concentrate all their attention on the body and fail to look at the patient as a whole. The number of patients whose malaise has a psychological basis, but is given an organic label, seems astronomical. If the symptoms are cardiac, the patients are said to have heart strain; digestive problems are diagnosed as some chronic "itis"; and even sexual problems are related to seminal vesicle inflammation or a tight vagina. Apparently the only somatic symptom not attributed to a bodily ailment is weeping.

Some doctors look at patients from a broader point of view these days, but medical schools still teach that before a patient can be considered neurotic, the possibility of organic disease must be ruled out. The ridiculous implication of this dictum is that if organic disease is discovered, the patient cannot be neurotic.

Most physicians would intellectually agree that the severity of all bodily symptoms is determined by the patient's state of mind as well as by the organic lesion. Pain is a case in point. One patient with rheumatoid arthritis will complain of endless torturing pain and be sunk in deep depression, and another patient whose joints are apparently organically similar will barely complain.

Physicians, aware of the type of criticism I have been leveling, strike back as did Dornhorst and Hunter, writing about holistic medicine in a recent issue of *Lancet,* a respected British medical journal.

Its proponents emphasize the distinction between the patient and his disease, and claim to treat the whole man, and to regard the patient as a person. They stress the frequency and educational importance of the more trivial disorders and their interrelation with emotional factors. There is an implication that much of the elaboration of modern investigation and treatment could be dispensed with if doctors were trained to acquire wisdom rather than to accumulate technical knowledge. Pervaded by an excessive belief in a unique therapeutic relation between doctor and patient, they aimed to substitute a pastoral role for technical care, which is assumed to be necessarily impersonal or even inhumane. This approach is often sympathetically received by laymen who are alarmed by various features of modern life, from divorce rates to sonic booms. They believe all would be well if doctors would turn their attention to prevention rather than care, and that medical students should learn more about health than about disease. The fallacy is a favorite with the amateur psychoanalysts who figure so prominently in left-wing journalism, and is also supported, for opportunist reasons, by some professional specialities, and by all manner of cranks and faddists. The essential superficiality, and indeed dishonesty, of this attitude is revealed when one of its advocates is faced with an illness in himself or in his family. The call then is not for the wise father figure, but for the man who knows most about so-and-so.

I plead guilty, in part, to the foregoing accusation. There are things I understand intellectually that I cannot yet deal with emotionally. Moreover, I take no exception to Dornhorst and Hunter with respect to patients with acute illness or gross lesions; scientific medicine is at its best with these ailments.

The gravest error of scientific medicine is the overvaluing of technology. We have already considered the errors produced by mystical medical machines. Another problem with technology is its overuse. Regardless of complaints, every patient of some physicians may routinely be subjected to a battery of laboratory tests. Extensive equipment-monitoring of patients is often done without seriously considering the benefits. Such procedures may be rationalized as defensive medicine against the possibility of a malpractice charge. Technology may be used to convince the relatives and the doctor of a very ill patient that, regardless of the outcome, everything possible has been done.

69

There is little doubt that the response of most doctors to other healers and folk medicine in general is attack in the form of ridicule or attempted exposure. Yet folk medical beliefs are strong and durable and the health professional who attacks them accomplishes little but the further alienation of his or her own patients.

Folk medicine is not founded on ignorance or a random collection of superstitious notions. It is a fairly well-organized and reasonably consistent theory of medicine. Folk medicine is rooted in time and tested by the experience of many generations, and its beliefs are tenaciously held. A record of success in treatment is taken as proof of validity; failure is rationalized or ignored. Sounds familiar, doesn't it? The true believers in metaphysical healing are literally impervious to attack, rational or otherwise. Their fervent belief is like a religion.

It is misleading to observe that a large proportion of the people who believe in the folk medical traditions of our culture are also receptive to scientific medicine. The patients who combine elements of both are perhaps wiser than the healers! It is the patients who constantly fit and adjust the new medicine to the old. There seems to be a growing population of patients in this country who have a better sense of the limitations of scientific medicine than do physicians themselves. It is likely that these patients learned the hard way.

The physician who convinces a patient that his or her illness is caused by germs will not alter the patient's metaphysical belief in the agent who put the germs there. It is not uncommon to see patients in a modern hospital receiving a folk healing treatment from a visitor.

There are patients who no longer give up their power in a passive healer-patient relationship. They blend folk and scientific medicine to enhance healing and create the effect of holistic healing. They assume an increased responsibility for their own well-being by finding ways to magnify their self-healing powers.

70

In *A Doctor's Dilemma,* George Bernard Shaw wrote that "Every profession is a conspiracy against the laity." Just as a major factor in the continuing reformation in law comes not from the legal profession but from juries, the energy for the growing reformation in modern medicine is coming from the patients. I have no doubt that healing can be more certainly and effectively attained if the treatment course is determined by a knowledge of metaphysical as well as scientific medicine. Only in this way is the treatment the closest possible approximation to the patient's own knowledge of what would be best for him or her.

Let me repeat once again my conviction that to function well the doctor would have to be a superbeing. In reality his obsolescence is manifold. His · education is archaic, with inappropriate orientations to both disease and people. The one-to-one physician-patient relationship and the fee-for-service economic arrangement are no longer functional. A physician's responsibility should be community-centered rather than patient-centered. The monopolistic, dogmatic role of the physician in patient care is the most dangerous dimension of his obsolescence. For all of these reasons, more and more of our citizens are seeking other types of healers.

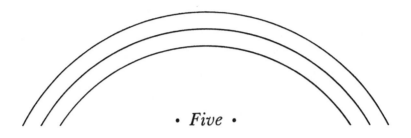

Five

The Mind-Body Connection

How would you answer this question: What is the relationship in a person between the mind and the body? It is obvious that we don't know enough about the answer if, like most people in our society, we see a physician for bodily illness, a therapist for emotional disturbances, and a clergyman for spiritual matters. Each time I have visited these separate professionals as an adult I have been at least vaguely aware of the fallacy of my action, but I knew no alternative.

Evidence of connections between mind and body is being presented to us continuously. I am aware of a connection at this moment. Several minutes ago I faced an empty pad of paper with the intention of filling it with the words you are now reading. This was preceded by my procrastination ritual, a period of pacing around the room to get my thoughts together. My thinking now is constantly interrupted by the apparent need to do dubious chores which somehow cannot wait: I make several trips to the bathroom, my straggly mustache needs trimming; I must sew on a button; and then the biggest delaying action of all—I must clean and arrange my large writing table.

When finally my body delivers my mind to the chair and

together we face the empty pages, I find I can't write. Finally, with patience, persistence, and a personal formula based on experience, all parts of me begin to cooperate and the words flow.

Something else just happened. During a break from writing I telephoned to cancel a tennis match I'd been looking forward to. I knew I didn't have time to go, but when my tennis partner answered the phone, I couldn't speak for a moment. No words came out. Eventually my disappointed emotions relented and allowed the negative message to be given by my voice.

There are so many examples of the tie between mind and body in everyday life. The way I walk when I'm high or low, my eye movements when I'm uncomfortable, my touch when I'm unsettled, and even my odor on a bad day.

Before we go too far into the difficult question posed at the outset, two other questions must be considered. What is a human body? What is a human mind? We're in such treacherous territory that a certain amount of cautious linguistic nitpicking is essential.

Your body is easiest to identify. It's the collection of flesh, bones, and organs which anatomists study and it is what the undertakers bury at the end of your life.

Your mind is what makes you different from other less interesting objects in the world like plants, rocks, and bodies of water. The differences are in activity, not in form. Human beings can do many things: jump, laugh, think, build, collide, and much more. A rock can only be acted on by an outside force or another object and roll, fall, or collide. Otherwise it merely exists. Our minds generate activities for our bodies that other objects cannot do.

Let's inventory the various capabilities of our minds: sensation, perception, analysis, memory, and belief; desire, purpose, intention, decision, and action; pain and pleasure, emotion and mood; and qualitites of temperament or personality, such as generosity, courage, and ambition. Quite an impressive list. 73

I've made a critical assumption to this point which now needs stating. The connection between mind and body has been assumed to be a relationship between two things. But is the mind a thing? When we say someone's mind is clear or talk about thoughts racing through one's mind, we are assuming the mind is a thing. The behavioral scientists take a different position. Their concern is how a person's bodily and mental characteristics are related, so they wouldn't speak of a mind-body connection but rather of a mental-physical connection.

Philosophers would raise a number of serious questions at this point, such as: Does each adult have one whole mind that nobody else has? Are all people alike so far as the relation of mind to body is concerned? Is the physical world a reality in which we can really know about our bodies? Such questions are mind-boggling, to say the least, and they lead to a dilemma: The human body is a material thing and the human mind is a spiritual thing, and although the mind and body interact, spirit and matter do not interact.

Going from the sublime to the ridiculous, let's discuss sweating. It is well known that emotion can cause some people to feel warm and finally even begin to sweat. The body's 'thermostat' for control of heating and cooling is located in the hypothalmus of the brain, a region where many of our most complex emotional responses are processed. We can speculate that during times of intense emotion the body's thermostat may be affected by the adjacent mechanisms. Signals go out to increase blood flow so that hot blood is carried to the outer layers of the body surface, which causes sweating, which in turn cools the body by evaporation. Sweating also occurs when the external environment is hot, when we have an infection, or even when we eat highly spiced foods.

Anatomically we know that we sense temperature through nerve endings located in the skin; however, the feeling that the skin is hot or cold may have very little to

74

do with the internal body temperature. Overexposure to the sun will cause the skin to be cool to the touch, while the body temperature may be over 100°. This homely example shows how many factors may be involved in a single body response.

So far we have been reviewing ideas related to the *involuntary* (or autonomic) processes that connect mind and body. The other side of the coin is the possibility of *voluntary control* over these same involuntary processes. The autonomic processes such as heart beat, breathing, and digestion have, in general, been the domain of scientific medical professionals. Many other professionals have been interested in helping us control voluntary activities such as behavior and diet. The possibility of control of autonomic processes fascinates both groups of professionals and a wide range of metaphysical healers as well.

Recently a man sat in the center of a brightly lighted room at the Menninger Foundation in Topeka, Kansas. An array of imposing electronic equipment was connected to his scalp, fingers, and forearms. Cameras hovered around him, recording his every move.

He dropped a six-inch darning needle on the floor, deliberately dirtied it by pushing it with his foot, then picked up the needle and unhesitatingly pushed it through the biceps of his right arm. The push required substantial effort and the observers saw the needle pierce the skin, penetrate the tough muscle tissue, pass through a vein, and come out the other side of the arm. The man did not flinch, looked nonchalant, and it appeared that he felt no pain.

As the needle was withdrawn, the physician in charge of the experiment asked the subject to cause his wound to bleed. On that signal, blood spurted from both sides of the wound, then stopped abruptly several seconds later when the subject said, "Now it will stop." In a short time the needle holes closed up, as if drawn by invisible purse

75

strings, and disappeared. When one of the observing physicians asked for a repeat experiment, but with no bleeding, the man painlessly complied. No amount of pressure on the arm near the needle holes could make blood appear.

We've all heard of yogis who can prance through burning coals or allow themselves to be stabbed by a sword. Now, there is a new breed of American mind-over-body people who allow themselves to be scientifically evaluated in well-known research institutes.

In the case I have been describing the man was intensely tested and observed and the possibility that he was some kind of mutant or physiological freak was ruled out. The climax to the testing occurred when an observing physician, inspired by the subject's confidence, decided to try the experiment on his own arm. The doctor started the needle into his own arm, froze, and sat there immobile. In the stunning silence that followed, the subject went to the doctor and pushed the needle through his arm. Later the doctor said he had felt nothing.

So to involuntary control and voluntary control of the mind-body connection we now add a third possibility, the role of *suggestion*.

Interest in the interaction of mind and body goes back to antiquity, but only in the early 1930s did this interest crystallize and become slightly legitimate within traditional medicine under the name psychosomatic medicine (PM). PM is the wide, gray, no man's land between the doctor who deals with bodily illnesses and the psychiatrist who works with minds. Today a professional journal is devoted to PM but it is not a medical specialty simply because not enough is known about it.

The causes of psychosomatic illness are still hazy and controversial. One view describes PM as "a group of disorders characterized by physical symptoms that are caused by emotional factors and involve a single organ system." Others believe that the bodily and emotional factors do not cause each other, but interact and influence one another and share equally in the illness. The never-ending issue of causality! After four decades of scientific research into PM there is some agreement that the personality and character development of the patient must be studied in order to understand the illness and determine an appropriate therapy. Getting to know and understand the patient is clearly a prerequisite for the physician when psychomatic illness is suspected.

In a later chapter on mental healing I will have much more to say about psychotherapy. The point here is that PM represents an uneasy marriage between scientific medicine and Freudian psychoanalytic concepts. I don't know whether to call it a shotgun marriage or a marriage of convenience; PM has elements of both. There is much evidence to indicate that the unsubstantiated theory upon which the Freudian analytic model is based would be little more than a historical curiosity if Freud and his followers had not themselves been physicians. Freudian ideas, now suffering the same slings and arrows that afflict other theories of traditional medicine, form a critical part of our medical establishment's approach to psychosomatic illness.

A young girl, aged sixteen, was a remarkable example of allergic skin reactions. She experienced occasional sudden swelling of her hands, face, and ankles during menstruation and under stress. Apparently the symptoms first appeared after she was hit by a car when she was fourteen.

Her medical history showed that at the age of five the girl had had both measles and chickenpox. At the time of her treatment for allergy she had a younger sister and three older siblings. The mother had appeared to prefer the younger sister, and, with intense jealousy and anguish, the patient had turned to her father for love and developed a deep attachment to him. She was now experiencing a recurring dream in which she had given birth to an illegitimate baby. In the dream her father would kiss her and then go away.

In mutual exchanges of irritation, resentment, and criticism between the girl and her mother, the skin symptoms were provoked. Later, during therapy, hives suddenly appeared before the doctor's eyes when the girl recalled feelings of abandonment and separation from her father. She was an attractive, exhibitionistic girl who constantly experienced intense erotic fantasies and seemed to have an insatiable desire for attention and love.

In essence, the skin of the patient had been transformed to a massive erotic organ. Lotions her mother had used after the measles and chickenpox attacks years earlier had greatly reinforced the normal eroticism of the girl's skin. When the girl was older and had headaches, her mother used loving caresses and compresses to give relief. As a young adolescent her desire to be touched caused feelings of guilt because of both the erotic sensations that were involved and the exhibitionistic drives she felt. According to her therapist, who worked from Freudian ideas, her symptoms were related to three emotional difficulties: childhood conflicts that she had carried over into adolescence, an apparent hereditary tie, and difficulty with identifying reality in her life.

This case offers one example of how psychosomatic illness is treated: the girl saw both a dermatologist and a psychotherapist for treatment of her allergy. If PM has any strength today it is as an amalgam of many specialties. Everything we know within the rational, scientific framework should be brought to bear on such strange illnesses.

Asthma is another illness that is interesting in this context. In studies of asthma, information is drawn from the fields of allergy, psychology, and social-epidemiological medicine. Thirty years ago bronchial asthma was poignantly described as "a child's suppressed cry for the mother." It was always suspected that asthma is related to emotional state. Three decades of study have revealed that the bronchial apparatus is constantly interacting with the environment while also being influenced by personal internal forces. Asthmatics readily show evidence of many powerful emotions, especially hostility. Choking off these negative impulses in order to get along in their world causes the asthmatic response. Or at least that's the theory.

When they discuss their work, philosophers of PM say that three broad areas are being scrutinized: the biological, the psychological, and the sociological. Only the spiritual has been omitted, probably unjustifiably. Results of research into physiological measurements are slowly becoming available, but in the area of psychological processes there is little that is new. We are limited by our lack of any real understanding of the physiology of emotions and our uncertainty about the validity of our knowledge of the psychology of emotion. The difficulty is that scientific medicine, with a backlog of information collected over a century, must blend with psychology, still the infant science of human behavior. The generation gap is too great.

Consider the problem of PM today. An understanding of the nature of this wilderness of illness requires a deep knowledge of a wide range of subjects about which we actually know little. The researchers who are contributing to our knowledge must function in the midst of a contemporary revolution against science and technology. Yet advancement of our understanding of PM offers the exciting possibility that scientific medicine will be able to deliver, in time, at least a partial version of holistic healing. Even now, scientific physicians aspire to make a "double diagnosis," that is, both an organic diagnosis and a personality diagnosis. But then what? There is no substantiated theory to merge the results and produce a general diagnosis.

Now let's consider further the subject of voluntary control of our organs and bodily processes.

Imagine the benefits if we could teach asthmatic children to expand the breathing tubes in their lungs voluntarily when they feel attacks coming on. It has always been assumed that bronchial tubes in the lungs expand and contract automatically and involuntarily. Like our heart beat, blood pressure, and blushing, our respiratory function has been looked upon as being beyond voluntary control. Now it has been shown that visceral "learning" can be achieved just as our skeletal muscles are trained to respond to signals from our brains.

I remember watching a friend of mine doing a strange exercise a few years ago. She sat for hours with her bare feet propped up in front of her. Patiently and sometimes frustratingly she learned to move her toes in complex patterns just like her fingers. "Opening up unused channels," she would say to me with a wry look. She is a member of a new community of people (young and old) who are discovering the bodies in which they live. Since we've worn shoes and walked on flat surfaces for millennia, the need for our toes to move independently has faded away. But the capacity is still there, along with capacities that we have never even dreamed of that lie dormant within us.

This subject has been given the provocative name *biofeedback,* and under that umbrella voluntary control of all types of what we have heretofore known as involuntary bodily processes is being studied and taught. Feedback is so natural to us that we take it for granted. It simply means monitoring what is happening and making adjustments. While driving, for example, we watch the position of the car with respect to the lane; and when we see that we are too close to either side, this information is processed by the brain, which initiates the muscular movements that turn the steering wheel in the appropriate direction.

A woman named Lois had experienced the misery of being unable to flex her neck and move her head for almost seven years. The doctors called it *wryneck.* The initial painful muscle spasms worsened until Lois's head was always pulled to the left. After trying everything that scientific medicine had to offer, Lois finally solved her problem by a method that involved sitting in a chair and responding to the clicks emanating from a box on a nearby table. Electrodes connected to a battery in the box were attached to the powerful neck muscle that pulled her head aside. The frequency of the clicking she heard was an indicator of the tension in that muscle. By means she can't explain, Lois learned to slow the number of clicks and release her neck. Once she had learned, she no longer needed the hardware but controlled the muscle spasm herself. It is frequently confirmed in research experiments that subjects are inaccurate in their reports on their own physiological states—that they are out of touch with their bodies. The clicking box supplied the information that Lois was not able to sense herself.

Today, all kinds of body signals can be monitored by special equipment that provides the feedback for an activity until we can provide our own. Skin resistance to tiny amounts of electricity, minute temperature changes, and electrical activity within muscles provide other ways of experiencing ourselves.

Some of the chronic ailments being treated experimentally with biofeedback include epilepsy, stroke paralysis, and back pain. Dr. Arthur E. Gladman, a California psychiatrist, reports that he has used biofeedback successfully to treat such disorders as migraine headache, Raynaud's Disease (a circulatory disorder), asthma, peptic ulcer, and chronic pain. His group of 175 patients ranged in age from eleven to eighty-four and all had specific ailments caused by some type of emotional stress. Dr. Gladman points out that the beneficial effects of his treatment went far beyond merely correcting the original physical complaints. He believes that the chief benefit of his experiment with the biofeedback technique is that it has helped patients control stress in general.

Stress is thought to be central to many ailments, and modern society is providing unprecedented levels of stress. When the patients develop a way to control internal forces, they develop a new awareness of self. It enables individuals to view the world in a new way.

"Biofeedback is the yoga of the West," said Dr. Elmer Green, head of the psychophysiology laboratory at the Menninger Clinic at a conference sponsored by the Academy of Parapsychology and Medicine. I like Dr. Green's metaphor because it points to a potential tie between scientific and metaphysical medicine.

Let's visit a biofeedback training session for a person who is experiencing chronic pain. The patient's pain is not related to any organic dysfunction and it literally defies medical analysis. The patient has been studied until some proxy measure of the pain has been determined; that is, body processes that change when the pain occurs have been identified. Such a change might be as simple as tension in some muscles or as complex as a temperature or blood pressure variation.

A device for sensing the proxy measure is connected to the patient, and a shrill unpleasant sound fills the room whenever the patient senses pain. The subject is told that the unsettling shriek is the pain and he has to turn it off.

Of the small number of patients in such experiments so far, about half learn to "think" the sound and the pain down to acceptable levels. It is exciting to realize that patients experiencing pain can wean themselves off drugs in this way.

At the Menninger Foundation eighty per cent of the migraine patients who have been treated by similar means have been relieved of their symptoms. The Menninger researchers' attack on this crippling form of headache was ingenious. They first discovered a relationship between the temperature of the patients' hands and the throb of their migraines. Patients were then taught to increase blood flow to their hands enough to raise hand temperature ten degrees in two minutes. As this happened, the patients relaxed, and as a frequent side effect their migraines were abated.

For some stroke and paralysis patients with brain injuries, whose normal feedback system has been disrupted, biofeedback instruments can serve as a substitute. The patient learns to monitor an activity through an undamaged channel. Imagine a blind basketball player shooting baskets by responding to a buzzer that goes off every time the ball goes through the net.

Biofeedback is attractive as a technique because the patient is in the driver's seat. He or she has not given up power but instead is developing it.

In recent years feedback has changed many of the physiological views previously held sacred by scientists. No panacea is being forecast by anyone, however, and the field is wide open to exploitation; the first cheap, exploitative, do-it-yourself equipment is already appearing on the market.

When we think again of the hold scientific medicine has on most Americans, it may be hard to imagine that the United States is providing the home for the biofeedback revolution in dealing with psychosomatic illness. We gulp down more pills to get rid of stress-related problems than any other nation in the world. High blood pressure due to abnormally high tension affects twenty-five million people in our country at present. Teaching us to relax is perhaps the greatest blessing that biofeedback training promises. The learning cycles of biofeedback are still mysterious and don't always work, but at the same time biofeedback doesn't appear to have any harmful side effects.

A proxy measure that has been highly praised as a means of combating our high levels of stress and tension is the alpha wave. Before describing alpha waves I must first go back to the discovery of brain waves shortly after World War I by Hans Berger, a German scientist. Since 1924 we have known that electrical activity can be detected on a person's scalp. From this there developed the speculation that these so-called brain waves are the result of electro-chemical activity in the brain cells. A seemingly magical machine called an electroencephalograph (or simply EEG) was invented to pick up these minute electrical signals by means of electrodes placed on the scalp. The tiny voltages are amplified by the EEG and are used to move inked pens on a moving strip of paper. There before our eyes is a measure of one miniscule function of that magnificent organ, the brain. But what do the random-looking inked squiggles mean? Regular cyclical patterns have been detected in the seemingly random brain wave variations. One of these, the alpha wave, recurs eight to thirteen times per second.

From various empirical observations, alpha has been associated with feelings of calmness, passivity, and relaxation. By monitoring the alpha as a proxy measure, the appropriate biofeedback equipment can help a person learn to relax.

Many people—both professionals and lay enthusiasts—have hopped on the alpha bandwagon, but brain waves are incredibly complex and are not yet well understood by anyone. There is still much to learn. Still, the identification and use of regular variations within the randomness of brain waves is promising for the future. Researchers have observed, for example, that alpha increases not only with relaxation but also with concentration, which opens up a whole new area of study and application.

The important question is: Does alpha produce relaxation or does relaxation produce alpha? Here again, causality is uncertain. More important, the question proposes its own alternative: After it has been *suggested* to a subject that he will relax if he produces alpha, he *does* relax and thereby produces alpha.

Dr. Ronald Melzack, an authority on pain, has found that it is not biofeedback alone that prevails over pain. Rather, pain is relieved by the distraction, suggestion, relaxation, and sense of control that are all part of the biofeedback procedure.

The placebo effect is another subject of great interest in our discussion of mind-body connections. It is a manifestation of our tendency to believe that we can make things the way we want them to be. I mentioned the placebo effect in passing in the last chapter with respect to testing new drugs. A great deal of experimentation has shown that placebos can duplicate both the positive and negative effects of drugs.

Folk literature on medical subjects abounds with accounts of sugar pills occasionally producing spectacular cures of otherwise untreatable illnesses. It is clear that in such cases some powerful social influence existed to effect the cure, or that spontaneous remission occurred.

Though the precise way a placebo works is not well understood, some clever medical practitioners have been able to put the placebo effect to work to help their patients. They have realized that the healing ritual is far more important than most scientific healers have ever allowed themselves to believe.

A story is told of an old painting in an Amsterdam museum. The painting was billed in all the local guidebooks as "the greatest painting of all time." The aesthetic experience of seeing the painting itself was essentially irrelevant after experiencing the massive placebo effect of the guidebook publicity, the multilingual signs, and the theatrical setting in which the painting was displayed.

Distance apparently breeds respect. It is said that no native of Lourdes, France, was ever cured by the shrine of the Virgin at Lourdes. The potential for influence is probably diminished by familiarity.

Respect for the source of the placebo seems to be one of the most important ingredients in its effectiveness. Cures by faith healers are based on the patient's faith in the healer rather than in what the healer says or does.

85

If respect for the placebo is diminished in some way, danger follows. There are documented cases of patients who were cured by new "wonder" drugs but had relapses when they heard rumors that the drug was ineffective.

In placebo therapy, the therapist gets to know the patient well enough to design what he calls a *placebo communication.* This fires up one powerful set of the patient's beliefs (his faith) to change another set of his beliefs (his problems).

Before going further into the subject of placebos we must recognize that a great many medical doctors vehemently oppose the use of placebos because of the alleged unethical aspects of the deceptive act. Yet there are many medical histories that show how the carefully concocted prescription of chemically inert preparations has dramatically alleviated many ailments, some severe, for which no organic causes could be discovered. If a placebo fails, no harm is done, and in most cases there will be renewed motivation to continue the search for the cause of the patient's complaint. When a placebo has been successful, on the other hand, careful follow-up generally is done in case psychological effects are masking organic disease.

We are not arguing ethics here, but rather examining a phenomenon. I cannot resist pointing out, though, that doctors who oppose the use of placebos often prescribe drugs at pharmacologically ineffective levels or for conditions that the drugs could not possibly improve. It is certain that fifteen milligrams of phenobarbital are no more a sedative than penicillin is antiviral. It seems that placebo-resisting doctors use inadequate active drugs and placebo-supporting doctors use inert drugs; either treatment may trigger a placebo effect.

The statistics of placebos are impressive. For about one suffering patient in three a chemically inert placebo cuts pain in half. In most cases the placebo is more effective if something active is added to give it a bitter taste or to cause it to produce a mild burning sensation.

Placebos with no physiological powers have soothed patients since antiquity. In medieval times the two most effective medicines were theriac powder, which included ground Egyptian mummy and viper flesh among its thirty to sixty ingredients, and the legendary bezoar stone, which was made from the gallstones of goats.

The French physician Armand Trousseau recognized in 1833 the implicit placebo effect in drugs when he said, "You should treat as many patients as possible with the new drugs, while they still have the power to heal."

A contemporary PM researcher, Frederick Evans, found that a placebo is 56 per cent as effective in pain relief as morphine, 54 per cent as effective as Darvon, and 54 per cent as effective as aspirin. Therefore, the placebo that is used as a substitute is effective in proportion to the strength of the painkiller that the patient thinks the doctor is using.

Regardless of the nature and quality of the healer-patient relationship, the placebo effect is always present to some extent. The active mechanism of the placebo, however, remains mysterious. Nevertheless, some of the conditions for a positive placebo response have been observed and they are worth reviewing.

Some degree of anxiety seems to be a prerequisite for the placebo response. Comparison of the pain responses of soldiers on the Anzio beachhead in World War II with that of patients with similar wounds in a civilian hospital offers a classic example. Both sets of patients suffered grievous but nonfatal wounds. The soldiers experienced much less pain and only one-third asked for medication to relieve their pain. The wounded soldiers were experiencing relief, thankfulness, and even euphoria at escaping alive from the battlefield. Their wounds meant they would be removed from combat. Their counterparts in the civilian hospital consumed large quantities of pain-killing drugs and worried constantly about the consequences of their injuries.

It has been shown in a great deal of research that fear or

anxiety increases pain. If both the patient and the healer believe in the therapy being given, their anxiety is lessened, and the placebo effect is stronger.

Enhancement of the placebo effect also occurs because diseases and the symptoms they produce vary in intensity in time and in different patients. For most diseases, the health of the patient and the powerful defense mechanisms developed through evolution mitigate the severity of the symptoms and eventually produce a cure. The development of a malignant tumor indicates the complete failure of normal defense mechanisms and placebo therapy probably wouldn't help. On the other hand, diseases with chronic remittent symptoms, such as the pain of rheumatoid arthritis, would be likely to respond to a placebo.

Positive placebo responses are much more likely when the central nervous system is being treated. Subjective responses, often based on parental attitudes and behavior, can be modified by placebo. Examples are temper tantrum, headache, nausea, vomiting, or postoperative pain. Good placebo responses are also frequent if the target of therapy is an internal variable under hormonal or autonomic control such as blood pressure, gastric acidity, or bronchoconstriction.

A final, but not yet fully understood, condition for a positive placebo effect is a direct healer-patient relationship, actual or implied. The prestige of a healer who is known to possess an array of wonder techniques will give a touch of magic to even the simplest interaction with a patient. Just being seen by such a healer is often enough to elicit a placebo response.

Still, even with our understanding of some of these favorable conditions, we do not know just what *causes* the placebo effect. Nor is it entirely clear which persons are likely to be reactors to placebos, although some researchers have observed that known reactors are outgoing personalities, are favorably disposed to hospitalization, are con-

88

cerned with visceral complaints such as constipation, and possibly are less emotionally mature.

On the other hand, certain generalizations have been revealed as untrue. The so-called suggestible person is not predisposed to placebo reactions, nor are women more likely to receive relief from placebos than men. A positive reaction to a placebo does not mean that the pain, discomfort, or disease state is only psychological and not organic. Conversely, a negative reaction to a placebo does not mean that the disease state is real.

Because its workings are so poorly understood, and because it is so often given for indefinite complaints, the placebo is frequently administered in an offhand fashion. It is usually assumed that the placebo response is a form of suggestibility or gullibility and that special care is not required.

Careful studies have failed to find any relationship between suggestibility or gullibility and actual sensitivity to placebos. Suggestion does play a part, however, in making the placebo *appear* more attractive initially or potentially more effective. It has been found that an injection is more impressive than taking a pill or capsule. If a pill is taken, a very large brown or purple pill or a very small bright red or yellow one will produce better effects than other size and color combinations.

Physicians generally understand that a placebo should be given only for definite purposes. The endpoint of therapy should be defined and the results of therapy should be carefully monitored.

The two most common situations in which placebos are used are in the treatment of diseases that have previously been effectively treated by placebos, and in the treatment of diseases for which there are no appropriate drugs but the patient nevertheless demands something tangible that can be interpreted as a treatment.

An example of the first situation is mild mental depression. It has been shown that mild mental depression will improve with any sort of pill, so it is reasonable to start with a placebo. A physician whose patient demands medication is often facing the choice between the deception of a placebo and the possibility of losing the patient to a colleague who may prescribe unnecessary and potentially toxic medication.

Healers of all types recognize that the placebo effect will be operating to some extent with every patient, but the wise ones know also that the direct use of a placebo will have a potential "toxicity" of its own. In the wrong hands, the placebo can be used as an appealing substitute for a difficult task of diagnosis. With this kind of uncertainty, it is fair to say that the placebo is treating the healer rather than the patient.

Believe it or not, the placebo can be habit forming. For example, the lives of some patients are made miserable by their compulsive conformity to an ulcer diet, which may have no definite effect on gastric acid production. Or worse, use of a placebo may actually foster the patient's conception that symptoms are due to physical causes when they are not.

A major point of this discussion of the placebo effect is that the healer provides the most effective enhancement of the placebo, but if the healer actually uses an inert substance, there is a risk of losing the patient's trust. A patient's discovery that he or she has been tricked into feeling better may cause new suffering and destroy the relationship with the healer.

An even greater danger to the patient exists when the healer is the placebo and makes an ill-advised chance remark or gives the appearance of preoccupation with something other than the patient, or raises an eyebrow or frowns at a critical point. Communication between the healer and the patient is rarely as good as it should be.

In a study having to do with routine surgery, one group of patients was exposed to standard hospital procedures, while a second group had, in addition, intensive contact with the anesthesiologist before and after their operations. The anesthesiologist discussed with these latter patients the nature and causes of normal postoperative pain. Though the two groups underwent operations of equal risk, the second group required only half the pain-killing medication that the first group did. The medication was ordered by the surgeons in response to patients' requests. The surgeons were able to release the patients in the second group 2.7 days earlier, on the average, than the patients in the first group. A most impressive example of how therapeutic intervention was certainly a placebo.

It seems clear that virtually every patient who sees a healer will be anxious and ignorant about his or her illness and about the mysterious treatment prescribed. Honest, straightforward communication almost always relieves anxiety. Better communication as a form of placebo might make fewer drugs and less toxic drugs necessary for relief of the patient's discomfort.

We can close this discussion of placebos by noting again that the limited circle of logic too often promoted by the modern scientific medical model is: Feel bad? You must be sick. Here's a prescription for a drug. The drug may provide symptom relief and/or a placebo effect, but the disenchantment of our citizens with the whole model is rampant. New settings that offer stronger placebos are being sought and discovered.

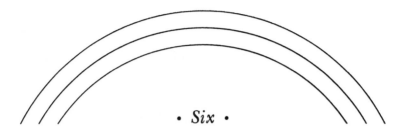

· *Six* ·

Alternative Medicine

Give yourself a test. What do you think of when you hear the words *psychotherapy, Christian Science,* and *naturopathy*? Do they make you think of *quackery, gullibility, superstition,* and *nonsense*—or do they suggest interesting possibilities outside of orthodox medical practice?

Accounts of patients' experiences with the many practitioners of so-called fringe medicine will be sprinkled liberally throughout the second half of this book. This chapter will list and briefly describe the scope and functions of a broad cross section of alternative healers and healing systems, or medical charlatans, depending on your attitude, and will serve as a glossary for the remainder of the book. The term *fringe medicine,* though frequently used, especially in England, gives a misleading impression. The alternative healing systems are not medically on the fringe of anything. Many do not have social acceptance but that is a different issue.

It is not a simple matter to separate orthodox medicine from fringe medicine. For one thing, traditionally trained physicians, once qualified, can practice any form of medicine they choose. There is a strange quirk in our society that allows a traditionally trained and legally licensed doctor to use healing procedures that would be illegal for alternative healers to practice. A few doctors actually use methods that are associated in the public mind with fringe medicine, and others, a somewhat larger number, are at least sympathetic to fringe medicine.

One obvious way of distinguishing fringe medicine from orthodox practice is to look at the formal educational requirements the healer has met, the principles behind the requirements, and the public licensing methods and standards that are applied at the end of the training. Or, more bluntly, we could ask about a healing system; is it taught in the standard medical curriculum?

No matter what terms are used or what tests are employed, a great gray area exists between orthodox and fringe medicine. Subtle gradations between the two have complicated my task in this chapter enormously. Where to begin? How to classify? What to include? My solution has been to use four categories. The first three, lists of practitioners, have been compiled according to their respective emphases on body, mind, or spirit. The last list covers those hybrid healers who belong outside or beyond the first three categories because they focus on two or more human dimensions simultaneously. The lists for each of the four categories are arranged alphabetically. I have deliberately and somewhat arbitrarily limited myself to a brief descriptive annotation for each listed subject. The reader who desires additional information will find a list of supplementary reading in the chapter references at the end of the book.

There were many dozens of possibilities for inclusion in the lists that follow, but I have concentrated on those alternative healing methods that are part of the patient-oriented medical revolution this book is describing, and on those that represent large classes of healers.

1. BODY

Acupuncture
This is a very old Chinese system of healing in which needles are inserted at certain meridian points that are mapped on the body. Diagnosis is done by taking the pulses. The method is sometimes used by American physicians but primarily as a painkiller.

Aikido
Aikido is one of the best known of the Japanese martial arts. Its basic principle is that motion is based on the flow of natural energy from a relaxed, centered person. Allowing the flow of natural energy is thought to have the effect of unifying body and spirit, thus helping to overcome sickness.

Air Therapy
This is more a point of view than a therapy. Those who hold it believe that good air is required for health and even more so for curing sickness. Various environments with different air conditions are considered conducive to healing particular ailments.

Alexander Method
This technique is based on the premise that the particular locations and times when people tense their bodies are directly related to illness. A course of retraining is given for relearning the natural use of the body, which presumably has been lost since childhood. The method is not merely a form of physiotherapy, but a demanding approach to a lifestyle that is said to enhance health.

Apple Cider Vinegar and Honey
This entry is primarily a tip of my hat to an allopathically-trained physician, D. C. Jarvis, M.D., of Vermont. His books *Folk Medicine* and *Arthritis and Folk Medicine* have

94

sold millions of copies. His folk-medicine healing is centered around the claimed curative powers of apple cider vinegar and honey.

Ayurvedic Medicine
This eastern healing discipline involves diet, herbs, natural medications, and Indian folk remedies.

Baths
Many types of water baths are used for both relaxation and healing. Examples are cold, hot, mineral, salt, foam, Turkish, scrubbing, inhalation, and jet baths.

Biochemics
In 1873, William Schussler, a chemist, believed that twelve salts are present in each human at times of normal health; and that ill health is related to an imbalance or absence of the proper salt combinations. After diagnosis, the biochemic tissue salts are given in amounts deemed appropriate to deal with the illness.

Breathing Therapy
Many fringe medicine systems involve the relationship of improper breathing to illness and low energy. Numerous breathing exercises have been developed with the intention of benefiting poor body conditions.

Chinese Remedial Massage
This massage focuses on regions of the head, neck, upper back, and spinal column. The intent is to balance forces of tension and compression in the body and in this way maintain good health.

Chiropody
Healing arts are applied to the feet. The condition of the foot is thought to be related to discomforts in other parts of the body, which are healed when the foot is healed.

Chiropractic

Bone-setting, as chiropractic was once known, dates from the earliest medical practice. Chiropractors treat partial dislocations of spinal joints that are thought to cause painful pressure on the nerves. Particular classes of illness are believed to be associated with these small dislocations. No drugs or surgery are used in treatments.

Color Therapy

Healing powers are attributed to colors. Each color is believed to be related to a set of physiological and emotional disturbances. The patient is irradiated with an appropriate colored light after diagnosis and drinks water that has been exposed to the same light.

Coué's Auto-Suggestion

When the earliest symptoms of an illness are apparent, the sufferer focuses the power of his or her mind on combating the illness by strength of will, imagination, and determination.

Dance Therapy

Movement and relaxation exercises are taught with the intention of loosening the body, improving body conditions, and increasing energy levels.

Diet

If you look, you can find one or more diets designed to ameliorate every conceivable human condition.

Earth Therapy

Healing is accomplished in this method by burying people up to the neck in various combinations of the earth's minerals.

Fasting

Many fasting methods belong to healing belief systems in

which the fast is intended to improve particular body conditions by helping the body eliminate specific toxic materials. Fasting might well be called the starvation cure.

Feldenkrais
A set of low-energy exercises is intended to correct body alignment and break old habitual physical patterns. The object is superior body conditioning and generally a better state of health.

Gravitonics
This exercise method is based on the use of a trapeze-like device. The assumption is that the weight of carrying one's body every day and other sources of tensions affect not only the muscles but the entire nervous system. Muscles are toned and tension is eased by exercises emphasizing the effects of gravity.

Herbalism
Herbs have been used since antiquity to treat symptoms of illness and to facilitate healing, but in the seventeenth century medicine and botany began to separate. Today herbalists claim that there is a suitable herb for combatting any disease the human body can experience.

Homeopathy
Hippocrates wrote in 400 B.C., "Through the like, disease is produced and through the application of the like, it is cured." A homeopathic physician operates on the principle that any substance that will cause a set of symptoms in a healthy person will cure the same symptoms in a sick person. More than 2,000 single-ingredient remedies form the homeopathic drug arsenal.

Hypnosis
The process of hypnosis is such that the patient responds favorably to most suggestions of the hypnotist, but usually

97

cannot recall afterwards how the suggestions were received. The sleep-like trance of hypnosis is used in psychoanalysis, in anesthesia, and in habit and phobia control.

Ionization
Research has shown that negatively charged particles called negative ions are conducive to a sense of well-being and have the capability of accelerating the healing process. Conversely, concentration of positive ions is detrimental to health. Negative ions can be produced by special equipment or experienced naturally in settings like the beach and at waterfalls. Proof is uncertain, but it is generally believed that breathing the negative ions or absorbing them through the skin facilitates healing.

Iriodology
This is a diagnostic technique based on disease identification by study of the spots that appear in the iris of the eye. The iris is divided into forty zones running clockwise in one eye, counterclockwise in the other. These zones are theoretically connected to areas of the body by nerve fibers.

Japanese Massage
Japanese massage is related to acupuncture. It depends upon manual manipulation of 365 acupuncture points on the body. Manipulation of appropriate spots in varying combinations is intended to treat such maladies and problems as asthma, allergy, diabetes, poor hearing, whiplash, bed-wetting, rheumatism, toothache, and mild depression.

Kneipp's Water Therapy
This is a school of therapy, practiced primarily in Europe, based on the supposed beneficial effects of cold water. Treatment includes water and air cures and the use of herbal teas. The cure technique emphasizes plunges in cold water alternated with physical exercise.

Lakhovsky Oscillatory Coils

This instrument is an example of the implementation of a phenomenon called *radiesthesia*. Oscillating magnetic fields are believed to have therapeutic effects. Small electrical currents are induced in the body of the patient to improve the tissue tone for a more correct, healthier vibratory pattern.

Lotte Berk Method

An exercise technique that combines ballet exercises, Yoga, calisthenics, and orthopedic exercises is used to improve muscle tone, body condition, sex life, and general health.

Massage

Among the many healing capabilities attributed to various forms of massage are relief of pain, stimulation of blood and lymph circulation, speeding the elimination of human wastes, reduction of swelling, lowering of blood pressure, and foremost of course, relaxation of muscles.

Mensendick System

This system stimulates impaired muscles into activity through will power. A series of exercises emphasizes keeping the joints of the body both tight and movable.

Moxibustion

Heat is applied to the body by burning herbs at some of the acupuncture points. As in acupuncture, diagnosis is done by taking the pulses and heat is applied at particular points for specific ailments.

Music Therapy

A sick person is defined as someone who has something wrong with his or her vibrational pattern. Appropriate sounds are found to adjust the vibrational pattern.

Naprapathy

In this system of treatment emphasis is placed on the gentle manipulations of ligaments and other connective tissue to restore a normal flow of energy in the body. Diet, vibration, and hydrotherapy are combined to restore balanced body chemistry. No drugs are used. Naprapathy has a natural kinship to chiropractic and osteopathy.

Naturopathy

Naturopaths are licensed to practice in seventeen states as this is written. They treat disease through the use of air, light, heat, herbs, nutrition, electrotherapy, physiotherapy, manipulations, and minor surgery. No drugs are used, and chiropractic is avoided.

Osteopathy

The osteopath is probably the most widely accepted of the alternative healers. Osteopathy emphasizes that the way illness occurs depends on the condition of the whole body and is not simply an isolated outbreak. There is a strong emphasis on the determination of causality of illness. Body manipulation is also practiced. The osteopath takes a course of study similar to that of the scientific physician and must pass the same licensing examination.

Phrenology

Phrenologists have a unique method for diagnosis of illness. They believe that there are links between certain kinds of unhealthy mental activity and nervousness, muscular weakness, and tendencies to sickness. The mental activity of a person is determined by studying the exterior of the skull and neck.

Phrenosophical Spiritual Healing

In this system, the healer meditates and asks for divine guidance in treating the patient. When the divine advice is thought to be received, colored silk is chosen and woven so as to enclose the unhealthy part of the body. The system appears to be a blend of spiritual healing, color therapy, and radiesthesia.

Polarity Therapy
This therapy combines elements of acupuncture, massage, manipulation, and yogic philosophy. The healer applies heavy pressure with thumbs, knuckles, or elbows to special points in the patient's body.

Radiesthesia (Radionics)
Vibrations in the patient's body are sensed by the healer in making diagnosis with this method, and vibrations are generated by equipment in the actual healing.

Reich's Orgonic Therapy
Wilhelm Reich believed that all muscle stiffness contains the history and meaning of its cause. He evolved a controversial orgone box to release stored stiffness of the muscle armor. These ideas are also the basis of Reichian Therapy in List 2, which follows on page 104.

Rikli's Sunshine Cure
What idea could be simpler? The sun is the source of all energy. Why not carefully tap that life-giving flow? Arnold Rikli thought that controlled sunbathing was a natural antecedent to good health.

Sauna
Bathing in fairly dry heat is alternated with plunges into cold water in this method. Colds, headaches, stiffness, pains, internal ailments, digestive disturbances and psychosomatic illness are apparently alleviated.

Sex Therapy
A mixture of techniques and exercises is used to improve the physical aspects of sexual functioning. Therapeutic

techniques have been developed based on material ranging from Wilhelm Reich to Masters and Johnson.

Shiatsu Massage
This is a Japanese massage which combines aspects of judo, spinal corrections, exercise, and finger pressure on body points to depress or stimulate energy flow. Relief is intended for asthma, rheumatism, slipped disc, headache, nosebleed, toothache, high blood pressure, gastritis, myopia, and the common cold.

Sleep Therapy
Sleep can be a therapeutic agent. A wide variety of bed and sleep environments are used to promote relief of particular ailments.

Spiritual Healing
Several types of healers call upon special energy sources both from within and without themselves in order to heal. Their patients are frequently those who have been given up by allopathic physicians.

Structural Integration (Rolfing)
A realignment of the body structure is attempted in this method by manipulation of the tough fibrous tissues that cover the muscles. As a result the body is in a more natural form and gravity is thought to be kinder so that many physical symptoms can be reduced or eliminated.

Tai Chi Ch'uan
This oldest of the Chinese martial arts is often thought of as meditation in motion. Basically it is a soft, flowing exercise form suitable for all ages. The intention is body harmony and good health.

Tantric Medicine
The central belief of tantric practitioners, who utilize a

102

kind of psychic healing, is that afflictions arise after a person is possessed by spirits. These spirits must be exorcised for healing to take place.

Unani Medicine
Herbs and nonorganic medications are applied after diagnosis, which is based on reading the pulses.

Vitamin Therapy
The use of vitamins as medicine is very controversial among physicians in this country. Nevertheless, many vitamin-oriented healing therapies have been developed to treat an extremely wide range of ailments, both physical and mental. Some therapies use only moderate dosages while others call for greatly exaggerated dosages.

Yoga
Hatha Yoga is principally concerned with the health of the body and the mind's successful mastery of the body. Its chakras (or centers of being) are similar to acupuncture points. Hatha Yoga emphasizes cleanliness, self-discipline, and vegetarianism.

Zen Macrobiotics
This diet has received much criticism in recent scientific studies. It is a low-water diet that stresses whole grains, fish, carrots, corn, and tea. The intent is to balance the Yin and Yang—the two opposed parts of a person. The ultimate diet is rice, which is alleged to cure all illness, including cancer.

And so we have the first list, Acupuncture to Zen. I have purposely not included any treatment or cure whose scope is extremely narrow, and I have not launched on the great sea of folk remedies. There are hundreds of books devoted to that rich mixture of historically successful methods of healing that have developed from old wives' tales, traditions, superstitions, and hunches. Folk healing activities have always been with us and still are, but they are not usually thought of as being a part of the healing phenomena we are discussing here.

The second list is devoted to healing of the mind. The term *fringe* has no real meaning here. Most therapies aimed at mental health have evolved in recent times; the oldest we have is psychotherapy based on Sigmund Freud's work. Freud invented the psychoanalytic wheel in 1895 when he published *Studies in Hysteria,* which became the cornerstone of his therapy. In the early years of the twentieth century a number of variations on the Freudian model evolved. The rate of evolution has accelerated since the 1950s. Today new models and new therapies are posited and dismissed at an astonishing rate.

This list includes most of the important psychotherapies that have come into being since Freud's time. Again, I have been ruthless in keeping the descriptions brief. To give us a common base before starting out, an entry describing Freudian psychotherapy might read: This traditional psychotherapy is based on a deep, prolonged, and tenacious analysis of the patient's complete psychic history. A cure of psychoneurosis takes place in the purging of repressed thoughts and emotions. There is enormous emphasis in the therapy on the impact of sexuality on a person's life.

2. MIND

Adlerian Analysis
Freud's associate Alfred Adler (1870-1937) did not believe in sexuality as the source of all human drives. Adler saw man instead as purposive, goal-oriented, and very much a social creature. The Adlerian therapist tries to win the patient's trust and to help him or her discover and magnify a sense of self-worth.

104

Alexandrian Analysis
This is a much shortened version of Freud's therapy that places emphasis on solving emotional problems through catharsis and abreaction. The analyst prescribes specific measures the patient should take to alter his or her life outside therapy.

Astrology
A system of accounting for life events based on the influences of seven planets. Interpretations, which attempt to predict stress situations that are likely to occur in a given week or month, vary according to the background, inclinations, and state of well being of the astrologer.

Auto-suggestion
(Developed by Coué; also included in List 1.) A self-hypnosis technique that is difficult to learn but when mastered can penetrate the unconscious imagination and serve to improve sleep habits, relaxation, and mental state.

Bach's Flower Remedies
Edward Bach (1886-1936), an allopathic physician, classified human mental conditions into seven major groups. One group is concerned with different kinds of fear. Specific flowers are ingested to improve a particular mental difficulty. Aspen would be prescribed, for example, if the fear was of the unknown, red chestnut for fear of other people, and rock rose for stark terror.

Bioenergetics
As in Reich's Orgonic Therapy (see List 1) muscular body armor is the point of attack in dealing with emotional difficulties. Stress exercises are used to release suppressed emotions. The therapist then provides an analysis of the emotional release that occurs.

Biofeedback Training

Biofeedback equipment (see Chapter 5) helps a person learn to relax and release tension. Since tension is related to mental stress, the general state of mental health should improve.

Client-Centered Therapy

Developed by Carl Rogers in the late 1940s, this therapy is based on personality development as being socially influenced, and the dynamics of neurosis as being socially determined. The therapy attempts to reduce the number of conditions that are necessary for self-worth and to increase concurrently the patient's self-regard. The role of the therapist is to be constantly sympathetic and encouraging.

Direct Behavior-Modification Therapy

This learning therapy tries to minimize a person's neurotic responses by means of talk therapy combined with the teaching of new responses. Behavior modification emphasizes present and future response patterns. New responses are learned by receiving reinforcing rewards. Failure to change elicits either no reward or punishment.

Direct Decision Therapy

Using talk to focus on the present aspects of an individual's behavior, the therapist probes for the inner decisions the patient lives by. Based on the premise that a self-induced, limited set of options has led to a neurosis, the therapy exposes new choices that will alter the behavior. Better decision-making by the patient should provide better personal insights and strengthen the resolve of the patient to make further good decisions.

Encounter Groups

An encounter group provides a setting in which complex interpersonal transactions are simplified by direct verbal and non-verbal expression and exchanges of feelings that are generated between members in that setting at any given moment. The intent is to strip away culturally conditioned verbalization so that the members operate at more fundamental levels of feeling and see their problems in the most basic coloration.

Ericksonian Analysis (Erik Erickson, contemporary Harvard psychologist)
The identity crisis is the central focus of this therapy, which is very faithful to the Freudian model. Empathy-sympathy techniques are used by a therapist who takes an active, guiding role. The term of therapy is much shorter than in conventional analysis.

est *(Erhard Seminar Training)*
est is a potpourri of therapeutic and human potential techniques, offered over two intense weekends, that attempts to dethrone intellectualization and emphasize feeling. It seems to attract many persons who would not consider other therapies, and by their testimonials, their lives are often enriched because they are made more aware of their feelings.

Existent Analysis
The nucleus of this analysis is the notion that all neurosis is grounded in the experience of being alive. A wide variety of techniques are used by the therapist in order to understand deeply how the patient perceives himself and his world at the present moment.

Frommian Analysis (Erich Fromm, 1900-   )
The Frommian analyst views the patient in the perspective of the whole of society. The patient is seen as an unwilling victim of the conditions of society. The therapist attempts to facilitate the patient's problem-solving from this point of view.

Gestalt Therapy

Personality is seen as the result of a process of continuous formation and destruction of perceived realities. Emphasis is placed on the patient's total self-awareness and awareness of others in the here-and-now. Incompleteness of personality impairs full connection between the patient and his or her environment and prevents a full awareness and spontaneity for living the present moment.

Graphology

Published texts on graphology date back to 1622, and it is a respected part of the psychology curriculum at many European universities. Handwriting is analyzed to pinpoint emotional and psychiatric problems. A connection between handwriting and disease has also been noted.

Group Therapy

Therapy groups are based on the therapeutic rationales of particular psychotherapies. The general goal of all group therapy is the changing of outlooks and attitudes. It takes time for an individual to develop the capability of talking about personal emotional problems in front of others. In the group setting exposure of personality and character continues until all persons in the group can see themselves as others see them and reconcile themselves to who and what they are.

Hornevian Therapy (Karen Horney, 1885-1952)

This therapy wears down patients' resistance until they acquire both intellectual knowledge and emotional knowledge of the specific ways in which pride is distorting their lives. In addition, the therapy re-educates patients to accept their real selves.

Hypnotherapy

The purpose of hypnotherapy is to recondition certain sensory reactions to the stimuli of anxiety so that physiological symptoms such as ulcers and headaches will not be produced. Habitual reactions of the patient are altered under hypnosis. After the therapist has changed the patient's anxiety-producing sensation system, the subject is trained in the use of the new responses in life outside of therapy.

Jungian Analysis (Carl Jung, 1875-1961)
The goal of Jungian therapy is to resolve disharmony within the psyche. The therapy begins with free association and dream analysis. That is followed by Jungian analysis of the patient's neurosis and by guidance of the patient toward normal functioning. Great emphasis is placed on dream interpretation.

Learning Therapy
This theory considers the symptoms of neuroses to be anxiety-avoiding behaviors. Neurotic symptoms are therefore considered to be learned behavior. Learning therapy restates or rearranges the elements of conflicts so that the related neuroses are relieved. The goal of the therapy is the correction of all of the maladaptive mental and emotional habits the neurotic person has learned.

Logotherapy
Victor Frankl, who developed this therapy after his experiences in German concentration camps, believed that the fundamental human motivation is striving to find meaning in life. Mental illness occurs when this motivation is frustrated. In addition to using traditional psychoanalytic techniques, the therapy requires that patients do exactly what they fear most. Patients' learned responses to the environment are replaced by more access to the richness of meaning that exists in themselves and in the things around them.

Maslovian Analysis

Self-actualization is the key concept in this therapy, which is based on the work of Abraham Maslow, a contemporary psychologist. It is assumed that in all of us there is an active, dominant desire for health. A hierarchy of the individual's needs is postulated, and the intensity of a neurosis depends on how far up in the hierarchy an unsatisfied need exists. The therapy attempts to lead the patient to self-actualization or the satisfaction of all the patient's needs.

Meditation

There are many different forms of meditation, but major goals common to all of them are relaxation and elimination of stress. Organic processes appear to slow during meditation and afterward renewed energy is usually available. A wide variety of techniques are used to clear the mind of all thoughts so that the true meditative state can be achieved.

Mind Power

Mind control teaches techniques that increase a person's concentration, will power, and intuition and lead to an increased ability to relax. These techniques are also used to cure insomnia and headaches, stop smoking and drinking, improve health, memory, and psychic ability, and enhance meditative states.

Palmistry

This is a 5,000-year-old method for which it is claimed that states of mental and physical health can be revealed by readings of the lines in the palms of your hands. The assertion is that palms change as health, intellect, emotions, and life experience change.

Paradox Therapy

This therapy is based on the assumption that neurosis and

110

psychosis develop in an individual as a result of contradictory information received, especially from parents, during childhood. The expression of neurotic behavior is encouraged so that it can be relieved. Hypnotism is used to produce neurotic behavior, and, as therapist and patient cope with the stimulated unacceptable behavior, new behaviors are produced.

Pecci-Hoffman Therapy (Fisher-Hoffman)

Group interactions are combined with supervised one-to-one therapy to purge neurotic behavior. Patients work alone much of the time, tape recording and writing a great deal under the supervision of a therapist. They relive their childhoods emotionally by writing detailed autobiographies that focus on the negative aspects of their relations with their parents. A spiritual teacher is also used at various points throughout the work. The general intent of the therapy is to transform life energy from negative to positive.

Primal Therapy

The assumption behind this is that each of us has accumulated a pool of pain since childhood because of unfulfilled or poorly met needs of that period. Attempts to deal with this pain produce neurotic behavior. The therapy encourages the patient to confront and experience the pain, even to the point of becoming overwhelmed by it, and then to scream it out without any control. It is hoped that in this way healing (the elimination of pain and neurotic behavior) will take place.

Rankian Therapy

Otto Rank, a defector from Freudian orthodoxy, considered the circumstances of a person's birth to be the underlying cause of mental-emotional disorders. His book, *The Trauma of Birth* was published in 1929. The pain, long repressed, of being separated from the mother's womb is

111

assumed to be the cause of any disorganization of the unconscious mind. In a free-wheeling exchange which is designed to shorten the usual term of therapy, every psychic complaint is interpreted according to the birth trauma rationale. The patient's will and psychic independence are strengthened by a highly supportive therapist until neurotic behavior has been dissipated.

Rational Therapy
The rational therapist believes that personality problems are created when the patient tries to live up to social and family standards. General psychotherapeutic techniques are used to show that the belief systems that stem from those standards get in the way of a rich life and obstruct the patient's ability to live rationally in the present. The major attractiveness of this therapy is in its emphasis on the present and its willingness to provide practical solutions to existing problems.

Reichian Therapy
The theoretical cornerstone of Wilhelm Reich, a neo-Freudian, was that character is the manifestation of a set of muscular armors which must be broken down before therapy can begin. When the armor is breached, emotional problems can be solved by harmonizing sexual energy. First, special exercises help to soften the body armor. Then techniques are used that enhance eroticism in an attempt to improve the quality of orgasm. Both sexual functioning and mental health are said to be improved. Reich's ideas were very controversial, and he died in prison in 1957.

Reikian Analysis
In Reikian therapy the first effort is to determine the type of mothering a patient has had to obtain a measure of the neurotic background. The quality of mothering is classified

in a system devised by Theodore Reik during the 1930s. The therapy proceeds from this classification, using standard psychotherapeutic techniques except that the therapist is more actively involved.

Scientology
Participation in the Church of Scientology promises success, improved I.Q., and better health (Scientology could have been included in the List 1), and, if that isn't enough, immortality. A form of questioning about events of the past is used in conjunction with mechanical measurements and interpretations of the responses. The cathartic impact of clearing past traumas from the subconscious by this means presumably raises the level of consciousness of the participant.

Sullivanian Analysis
Harry Stack Sullivan was an advocate of the idea that cultural factors are the fundamental causes of neurosis. He saw failures interpersonal relationships as the crucial function of neurosis, and decided that therapy must be an interpersonal process. In this therapy, the therapist is deeply involved and provides a vigorous source of new psychic influence to the patient, who, through a series of steps with the therapist, unlearns neurotic behavior. Reik's book *Listening with the Third Ear* (1948) presented the principles.

Transactional Analysis
Eric Berne constructed a therapy intended to be simpler and more easily interpreted than the Freudian model. The TA model is based on each person possessing behavioral patterns identified as *parent, adult,* and *child.* The person is analyzed in terms of characteristics of these patterns.

Yoga
The word Yoga means union and suggests the integration

113

of mind and body. Through meditation, exercise, and breath control, the mind and body are brought together in harmonious action. The aim of Yoga is to establish one's equanimity under all circumstances.

As I am sure you already realize, cataloging the many healing activities is a most difficult task. Perhaps I have omitted your favorite or you may feel that an activity such as Yoga could be placed on all of the lists.

In any case, let us pause and review our progress. List 1 covers healing activities in which profit to the body is dominant, although some entries also specified claims of benefits for mind and spirit as well. This is a good place to remind ourselves that our model of the four dimensions of man is just that—a model. The labels body, mind, emotions, and spirit are convenient cognitive devices that allow us to discuss incredibly complex matters, but the model's relationship to the reality of being is not as sure a thing as may have been implied. Bear in mind that it is unlikely that there is a body/mind separation, and also be aware that we are dealing with *effects* which *appear* to emanate from either a body source (sensations) or a mind source (thoughts). These appearances allow us to make an intellectual separation.

The healing methods in List 2 are aimed at emotional problems, but sometimes the body is involved too, and a high potential for mental and spiritual development is suggested in a few listings.

The third list, which follows, has a spiritual focus. My criteria allow me to include both techniques that are spiritually stimulated and techniques that are aimed at spiritual development. This is perhaps a bit confusing, but it is in the pursuit of simplicity. Because there is no generally accepted vocabulary for discussing spiritual healing, I have tried to make each entry as self-explanatory as possible.

114

3. SPIRIT

Absent Healing
This is a form of spiritual healing in which the patient is not present at the scene when a healer or a group of healers works toward a cure. A photograph, description, or personal possession of the patient is used as a stimulus. Spiritual energy is focused by the healer to cause physical healing of the patient.

Catholic Healers
The Roman Catholic faith has been the stimulus for healing both at sites, such as Lourdes, or with objects, such as the relics of a saint. The Church subjects these healings to careful and lengthy scrutiny before accepting them as "miracles."

Cayce, Edgar
This American psychic (1877-1945) healed by prescribing unorthodox and often complicated therapies. His diagnoses were accomplished while he was in deep trances. It is not clear whether the source of Cayce's diagnostic knowledge came from his mind or the patient's mind. Several organizations have continued to promote his principles and approaches since his death.

Christian Science
As a religion, the Church of Christ, Scientist bases its approach to healing on the conviction that mind is God, and, since man is made in the image of God, who is perfect, illness is conceived of as an error. Since they consider the origin of all disease to be mental, Christian Scientists avoid drugs, doctors, and hospitals. This is an example of faith healing at its best.

Contact Healing
The physical contact of a spiritual healer is intended to

115

provide a path for a flow of healing energy from the healer to the patient. Some healers insist that they act only as channels and that the healing power comes from a higher source. Many patients experience the sensations of heat and tingling when contact healing is occurring.

Eckankar
A movement founded by Paul Twitchell in 1965 which purports to heal by *soul travel* or by mail. It is a part of a general spiritual movement which vaguely seems to resemble Yoga.

Enlightened Healing
A healer who functions because he possesses special mystical knowledge or cosmic consciousness is said to be *enlightened*. This type of healer often heals while in the meditation state.

Evangelistic Healing
When healers have intense charisma and power of personality that they combine with a theatrical or religious setting, I call them evangelistic healers. Well-known examples are Kathryn Kuhlman and Oral Roberts. They appear to heal by convincing people that they can heal.

Spiritualists
Spiritualists have generally been thought of as being mainly interested in communicating with the spirits of the dead. Recently, however, some spiritualists have promoted the practice of healing the mind, body, or spirit by means of prayer, meditation, laying on of hands, manipulation, and the like, whether or not in the actual presence of the patient. A major distinction of this type of healing is that spiritual teachers are used to dictate the type of treatment.

Radiesthesia
More than any other method of healing listed here, Radies-

116

thesia has been the target of ridicule and antagonism. The healing is an attempt to apply to medicine the techniques used in water divining. The healers use a variety of equipment to help them sense the location in the body and the nature of the disorder. Physical distance between healer and patient is apparently of no importance to the healers.

My list of spiritual healers is likely to generate controversy among knowledgeable readers simply because there are no generally accepted categories or labels. In this connection it is interesting to note Brian Inglis's observation that the miracles of Jesus can be classified in seven categories, which also would apply to the healers described in List 3:

1. Healing by contact.
2. Healing by contact using accessories.
3. Healing by command, with or without accessories.
4. Healing by release from any guilt.
5. Unpremeditated healing.
6. Healing at a distance.
7. Relegated healing.

The subject of this book is holistic healing, yet, as we have seen, we do not possess the knowledge to heal the total person. At best, we make selections from the assortment of the three lists, and try to combine these healing efforts with those of the traditional physician to simulate whole-body healing. Such a mixing of healers has to be based on the awareness, intuition, knowledge, and luck of the patient.

As an idea, nothing could be more attractive than a synthesized healing procedure intended to work with combinations of body, mind, emotions, and spirit. Not just one element per practitioner or program, but more than one. In a way this is a specious idea; again, our model of the four dimensions of human beings may get us into trouble.

117

We must keep in mind that it is impossible to develop one part of a person without having impact on all parts. The potential value, however, in the pursuit of coordinated therapies is the possibility of developing the holistic idea for the future.

The new breed of holistically-minded patient has no models to observe. We have no generation of people who have grown up with a deep awareness that total health means spending a major portion of their life energy in developing body, mind, emotions, and spirit in mutually reinforcing ways.

When any healing program offers direct coordination or enhanced development of multiple dimensions of being, it is sure to be an attention getter. My last list is one of such hybrids and is quite short. Some of the listings that follow will repeat healing activities that appeared on one or more of the first three lists; others will be new. Some are programs or organizations that actually synthesize many practices for you.

It is not uncommon to find individual healers who attempt to combine many of the healing practices of the previous lists. They literally offer a smorgasbord of healing according to their own unique talents and inclinations. I have chosen not to attempt a list of such individuals.

4. HEALING HYBRIDS

Arica
Body, emotions, spirit. Arica is based, in part, on the Sufi tradition, which employs exercise, breath control, chanting, and meditation.

Astrology
Body, mind, emotions, spirit.

Bioenergetics
Body, emotions.

118

est
Emotions, spirit.

Faith Healing
Body, emotions, mind, spirit. Examples are given in List 3.

Gurdjieff
Body, emotions, spirit. Centers have been established where the work of the Russian mystic Gurdjieff is used. Body-movement work is blended with psychological exercises and prayer.

Mind Power
Body, mind, emotions, spirit.

Neo-Reichian Therapy
Body, emotions. There are a number of variations on the basic Reichian theme, all focused on breath control and reducing the body's muscular armor.

Pecci-Hoffman
Emotions, spirit.

Psychosynthesis
Mind, emotions. Psychosynthesis begins with each person's current situation as she or he perceives it. A variety of activities are blended in an attempt to harmonize the many, often conflicting, elements of a person's inner life. Examples of the techniques used are guided imagery, journal keeping, intuition development, and training of the will.

Scientology
Body, emotions, mind, spirit.

Yoga
Body, emotions, spirit.

Zen

Mind, emotions, spirit. Zen is basically the practice of observing. The objective is to live life as an interesting experience without attachment. This leads to learning about your true nature, which is possible only after your mind has become open to every experience. The fundamental Zen practice is an eyes open, "just sitting," form of meditation.

We have now been through a supermarket of healing activities. Shamanism, voodooism, and the like have not been included in this chapter because they seem inappropriate to the American healing scene this book is examining. Some readers may point out that I have included some growth activities, and that is true. In most cases separating growth from healing is not feasible.

In the next four chapters we will explore the actual experiences of persons who by interesting means have become involved in some or many of the healing activities of the four lists and have created their own personal forms of holistic healing, with impressive results.

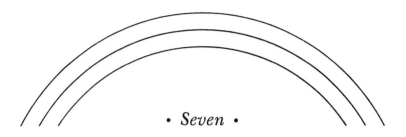

Seven

Healing the Body

In the preparation of this book I have talked with many people about their health habits. Most of the people I've interviewed are ordinary people whose lives do not contain elements that would identify them as famous, rich, or bizarre. What they have in common is a desire to live in this world in the best possible personal and social state.

That phrase bears repeating: the best possible personal and social state. It states my sense of what a mixed group of people were trying to say to me. The meaning that phrase conveys is one of harmony. They have the wish to live a life with a natural harmonious balance between their being and the world they live in. My focus in the interviews emphasized the role of health, of course, since a person's health is a fundamental element of living harmoniously. Every environmental factor affects our health and in turn our state of health influences everything that happens to us.

The interviews presented in this chapter show how different people are experiencing holistic healing in their lives. Each of the interviews acts as a springboard to a more detailed discussion of some of the healing methods used.

121

I'll start with Louise because her style of health care is based on a blend of homeopathic and allopathic medicine. Louise is an attractive, vital, seventy-five-year-old woman. She has a firm, warm handshake, good eye contact, and wastes no time with chit chat.

Louise has been a widow for two years, and prior to her husband's death her life was spent as a traditional middle-class housewife. She had a close relationship with her husband and emotion creeps into her voice when she talks about him. His death came after a series of progressively more damaging strokes. The attending physician throughout this period was chosen because he had a reputation for allowing elderly people to die gracefully. It was understood that there would be no excessive prolongation of a hopeless condition. Louise's husband made it clear that he wanted the responsibility of his own death, and Louise backed him up when he was too weak to speak for himself.

In addition to her role as wife and mother, Louise was deeply involved in church activities and community services. She proudly displayed political reports she had researched for the League of Women Voters, and read me excerpts about her religious convictions from her personal journal.

Louise may sound like someone you know. I think of her as a salt-of-the-earth woman. She has always been healthy and attributes her good health to careful eating and to keeping busy and involved. Her relationships with physicians have been generally satisfactory, but she often followed her own intuitions when she felt they didn't know what they were doing. As Louise aged she became aware that her family doctor had less and less to offer her, and her connection with him nearly disappeared.

A few years ago, through her community service work, she was approached by some therapists who wanted to form a therapy group for elderly people. Louise located the people for the group and joined it herself. The group was extremely free in form and Louise had many new experiences. The members learned to speak openly about their lives and to share their experiences and knowledge about growing old and life in general. Physical exercise was also a part of each meeting. Bodies that had moved only minimally in recent years began to stretch and bend gently in search of long-lost tone.

The group leader's main effort, however, was to encourage the participants to become aware of themselves by speaking openly about their feelings and learning to relax. Louise enjoyed the group tremendously. They laughed constantly, she told me, and had fun.

So many of her own experiences regarding health and old age were reinforced by the group, and new ideas were added. Topics such as diet, sex, exercise, aversion to drugs, loneliness, pain, relationships, health, death, shyness, rejection, and fears of every kind were openly discussed.

Among Louise's many new experiences was biofeedback training. She learned how her body tension increased the pains of aging. The biofeedback equipment assisted her in relaxing by monitoring her breathing exercises and measuring her alpha waves. In time the equipment was no longer necessary. When the process of aging caused aches and pains, Louise found that her relaxation exercises made the discomfort much more tolerable.

Her reaction to a recent accident sums up her attitude toward health and shows how she practices a form of holistic healing. Louise broke her hip. This is a common injury among the elderly, and is greatly feared because of the long term of healing required and because of the possibility of a shortened leg after healing.

Louise's approach to treating her broken hip was definitely holistic. She located an orthopedic surgeon who was noted for using the latest methods and equipment, and who advocated the shortest period of confinement. During the period immediately following the accident—in the hospital and later in the convalescent home—she used her breathing exercises to help her relax and to lessen the pain.

123

She had friends bring her food to supplement or replace the hospital diet when it was inadequate. Other friends gave her massages to help relax her body. Louise received polarity therapy treatments in the hospital, and she began taking a natural homeopathic medication known for its ability to promote the mending of broken bones.

In short, Louise took charge of her own recovery. She used her own self-awareness, and asked for the treatment she wanted. She was straightforward with her doctor and let him know when she was not getting the results she wanted from his prescribed treatment. While her hip was mending, Louise continued with her own physical exercises as much as possible, to maintain her body tone.

From Louise's story let's select one thread and expand it into a little healing Chautaugua. She used the best aspects of allopathy and homeopathy to facilitate natural healing. We need at this point to look more closely at homeopathy.

Homeopaths and allopaths are like Republicans and Democrats. Any idea generated by one group is generally rejected immediately by the other group, regardless of the merit of the idea. This is bad policy; many medical difficulties that our traditional allopathic doctors face today are solvable with homeopathic ideas. Immunization against disease stands today as a pillar of allopathic practice, yet it is a homeopathic concept.

In 400 B.C., Hippocrates wrote, "Through the like, disease is produced, and through the application of the like, it is cured." Homeopathy was founded on this principle in the early 1800s by Samuel Hahnemann, a German allopathic physician. Two other homeopathic principles evolved in time: the use of a high potency microdose and treatment of the patient rather than the disease.

Hahnemann was appalled at the brutality and inefficiency of the allopathic medicine of his time. His experiments with drugs that produced certain illness symptoms in humans convinced him that those drugs could be used to cure a wide range of diseases that presented the same symptoms.

Hahnemann rigorously tested his chemicals on healthy people before he tried them out on the sick. In this testing he moved away from the allopathic approach and formed his drugs as single uncompounded natural substances which were given in minute doses. He found that the weaker the dose, the more effective was the remedy.

Some critics charged that the dilution of the original homeopathic chemical was so substantial that only a placebo effect was operating. While most allopathic physicians merely disliked homeopathy, chemists were violently opposed. They saw their financial ruin in the tendency of homeopaths to prescribe simple chemicals in small amounts.

The third principle of homeopathy, and to me the most attractive, requires that the nature of the patient be considered in conjunction with the nature of the disease. It seems patently clear to homeopathic physicians that each patient has a different heredity, constitution, and temperament—factors that could influence the nature of the disease. A detailed knowledge of the patient is a prerequisite to treating an illness, as well as preventing it.

Philosophically, Hahnemann was far ahead of his time. He believed that illness can itself be a form or phase of cure and should be studied carefully rather than mindlessly attacked; symptoms were to be given attention rather than simply removed.

Homeopathy could have become a strong ally of allopathy, but it didn't turn out that way. The idea of introducing an offending substance into a system to desensitize it survives only in vaccinations and allergy shots in conventional allopathic medicine today.

Hahnemann was persecuted by the traditional medical establishment most of his life, but his ideas took hold throughout Europe and in the United States. In cholera

125

outbreaks during the mid-1800s the death rates in homeopathic hospitals were half those found in their allopathic counterparts.

Early in the twentieth century, however, the much publicized triumphs of the drug industry and the unflagging opposition of orthodox medical establishments caused the homeopathic movement to shrink to miniscule size. By 1975, only eight homeopathic physicians were listed as practicing in the New York City area and even Hahnemann Medical College in Philadelphia was offering homeopathy only as a post-graduate summer course. Brian Inglis writes of the recent state of the homeopathic physician "as a poor relation, eccentric and embarrassing, but still loved by some of the best people, which makes it difficult to treat him with the contempt he deserves. He has, however, learned to live quietly within the Establishment, in a small room in the East Wing: at least the best people have taught him how to behave in society. Anyway he can't live forever. . . ."

Well, maybe. Louise has discovered homeopathy hidden away in the East Wing. She likes its holistic view of the patient, and a growing number of patients feel the same way. The homeopathic physician is making a modest comeback.

Homeopaths use the same laboratory tests and x rays any doctor might use, but they also investigate the patient's personality and mental state. Special attention is given to examining patients' diets, and to the way patients describe their sensations.

You will recall from Chapter 4 that it was Pasteur's germ theory that was most influential in halting the spread of homeopathy. Homeopaths believe that microbes are not the cause of disease. Instead they are more like looters in a city where law and order have broken down. They appear after the trouble. Arresting and shooting the looters will not save the city. Law and order must be restored—or so the homeopaths put it—by reviving the life force.

126

Many children contract tuberculosis and polio in such mild forms that it is never noticed. An allopath might say that only in innocuous strain of bacilli was involved, but a homeopath would counter that certain people simply are not prone to these diseases. More articles in current medical journals are beginning to support the view of the homeopath. The critical issue at stake is research. The emphasis should change from concentrating on identifying and destroying the bacilli, to determining why certain people are immune.

An emerging factor that is changing the status of homeopathy in the public mind is the growing concern over drug side effects—iatrogenic illness. Homeopathic medication rarely produces side effects because of the miniscule doses that are prescribed.

The other side of the coin, however, is the question of whether those tiny doses can do any good. Allopaths often assume that no demonstration of the effect of minute doses has ever been shown, but this is not correct. Orthodox medical and scientific literature abounds with examples. For instance, when iodine was found to be essential to health, it was added in small quantities to the diets of people in the form of iodized salt, while the bottle of tincture of iodine from the drugstore was correctly labelled poison.

Some biologists contend that small doses of drugs encourage life activity, large doses impede it, and very large doses destroy it. The homeopaths, however, do not have concrete research results that prove their microdose really works. The double-blind tests used in testing allopathic drugs cannot be used because they are based on the assumption that, on the average, different people react to like amounts of the same drug in the same way. A homeopathic physician is likely to change the dosage or content of a prescription when the patient's mood changes, so double-blind tests have no meaning.

We live in a culture that seems to believe that more is

better, and anything to the contrary will have to be carefully demonstrated. Yet we are living in a time when allopathic ideas are declining in popularity, and patients are rediscovering homeopathic principles. Perhaps this will lead these two antagonists to become allies, finally. The two medical viewpoints have complementary aspects and could reinforce each other in a marvelous blend.

Another alternative healer who is attracting a new kind of patient is the chiropractor. Formerly sought out by old folks, poor people, and eccentrics, the chiropractor appears to be on the verge of beginning a new era of acceptance and activity.

Jim is a holism-seeking patient who is a recent convert to chiropractic. He is becoming involved in holistic healing by developing a network of alternate healers, including a chiropractor. His discovery of what a chiropractor had to offer him was actually an accident, and I will set the stage for a discussion of chiropractic by recounting his story.

Jim has problems with his lower back. The main reason for his involvement with alternate healers is his back trouble. The lower back is a murky, hard-to-diagnose, problem area for many healers. A psychotherapist will mutter claims that the lower back is the physical location of emotional difficulties. A physiotherapist will label the lower back as the physical hinge of the body and emphasize that the mechanical load it carries requires constant attention in the form of specific daily exercises. And on and on. Entire books are written on the subject of lower back trouble and each healer has a different viewpoint.

Jim went through a number of healing options in the belief that each had some measure of validity. He reduced the tension in his life, exercised each morning, worked on his emotional limitations with a therapist, meditated, was careful with his diet, and generally focused a lot of self-awareness on his body, especially his back, to see what he could sense for himself. It all seemed to help. Jim's general health improved, and his back seemed to be less troublesome. Every now and then, however, it would go "out." Every six months or so his lower back became very sore, and, in spite of all his efforts, took several weeks to get back to normal. When his back was extremely painful, Jim would see a doctor who would invariably prescribe a muscle-relaxing drug to quiet the muscle spasms he could detect in Jim's back. Symptom relief was all the physician could offer. Using a drug was undesirable to Jim, but no alternative was known to him at that time.

One year while Jim was on vacation in an isolated rural area a strenuous tennis match (that's a guess; Jim is never sure of causality) left his back undone. Cut off from his usual health sources and almost immobilized with pain, he asked for help from a local resident. The neighbor immediately arranged an appointment with a nearby chiropractor for later that day. Although he was hardly in a position to argue, Jim nevertheless continued asking around, but everyone in that small community gave the same answer. "See Dr. James, the chiropractor."

So he did, and a new member was added to Jim's holistic healing team. The visit began with Jim providing a complete medical history and a detailed discussion of his complaints and sensations. After a careful examination by the chiropractor, an x ray was taken.

While the x-ray film was being processed, the chiropractor began a special massage of Jim's back. Jim had received many different massages, but this one was new. He was put on a special sectional table where wedges and cushions were used to move parts of his body to certain positions. These movements were followed by rest periods to "let gravity do its work."

Jim's body had become distorted from coping with the back pain. When the chiropractor slowly moved him back to a normal posture the massage quieted the muscle spasms and relaxed the tension in the overstressed muscles.

As Jim lay quietly while the chiropractor went to get

the x ray, he realized the pain was gone. He felt relaxed and as if he were floating in the aftermath of the massage. There was still a sensitive spot in his lower back, but it didn't bother him much as long as he was quiet and stayed relaxed.

Jim and the chiropractor spent a lot of time going over the x ray together. By examining the picture of Jim's spine, Dr. James was able to make perceptive comments about Jim's body and to ask a particularly important question. "Do you realize that you stand on your right leg a lot of the time?"

Jim was shown the spot on his lower spine, where, the chiropractor suspected, a minor misalignment was causing the pain. After explaining what he was going to do, the chiropractor adjusted Jim into a twisted position on the table, made a quick levered movement, and Jim heard a loud pop as all his breath whooshed out of his lungs.

As Jim told the story of his rapid recovery to me he said, "That man spent over an hour with me and he has the sensitive touch of a healer. As I was leaving his office he looked in my eyes for a moment and said, 'Try not to take life so seriously'." Jim felt this was in incredibly perceptive remark.

I have talked to a number of people who regularly see a chiropractor to complement the services of a traditional physician. These are thoughtful patients who know what they want and they seem to get it from a chiropractor. They are especially enthusiastic about the physical contact and the long unhurried appointments. I have also collected many readings from the health and medical literature about chiropractic. Some of the titles speak for themselves: *The Ghost and Hoax of Chiropractic Licensure, The Right and Duty of Hospitals to Exclude Chiropractors, Healthy Quackery: Chiropractic, Inevitable Decline of Chiropractic,* and Ralph Lee Smith's book, *At Your Own Risk.* An astounding number of negative articles about chiropractic are written by allopathic physicians, who

130

charge that chiropractors have never devoted any effort to validating their theories, that instead chiropractic has expended its time, energy, and money in justifying its existence. Doctors claim that chiropractors add to *their* load because the doctors must pick up the pieces and repair the damage done by the chiropractor either directly or through delaying of proper medical care.

Modern chiropractic was born in 1895 when Daniel David Palmer hypothesized that the condition of the spine is central to good health. Body manipulation techniques have appeared, however, in all of recorded medical history.

At the onset of chiropractic, Palmer took credit for curing one patient of deafness and another of heart trouble, by manual adjustments of their vertebrae. On the basis of these two cases, Palmer concluded that a partly dislocated vertebra is the cause of 95 per cent of all diseases. Students of anatomy then and ever since have taken exception to Palmer's conclusions. As we have seen in Chapter 3, however, scientific verification as a credential may have little to do with actual healing. In a patient-healer relationship it is *belief* in what is happening that generally facilitates healing.

Today the estimated 16,000 active chiropractors in the world are divided into two, often bitterly opposed, groups. The International Chiropractors Association, represents the so-called "straights," who regard any form of treatment other than spinal adjustment as a heretical deviation from the doctrines laid down by the founder. The "mixers," represented by the American Chiropractic Association, augment their spinal adjustments with nutritional supplements and with some forms of physiotherapy. The two groups agree only in renouncing the use of all forms of medication, vaccination, and surgery.

In spite of the defensive, often self-righteous, and sometimes even vicious attacks of physicians, who at best dismiss chiropractors as sophisticated masseurs, a growing number of physicians not only refer patients to them, but often secretly utilize chiropractic services for themselves and their families.

When teamwork and goodwill exist between doctors and chiropractors, the patient generally benefits. A woman who thought her chest constriction and breathing difficulty were symptoms of "housewife's backache" saw a chiropractor and was twice referred to doctors—once to an orthopedic specialist and the second time to a general practitioner. Cooperation among the three healers helped the woman recover—from asthma.

How does one become a chiropractor? To be accredited by the Council of Chiropractic Education, a chiropractor must have a minimum of two years of pre-professional college credits and pass a four-year residency course in a chiropractic college.

In the United States chiropractors can be licensed in every state except Louisiana and Mississippi. In most states, licensed chiropractors can treat infectious diseases, examine school children, sign health disability and death certificates, and treat a wide variety of nervous, digestive, and circulatory disorders. In spite of these license options, hospital privileges have been denied chiropractors.

Nineteen states now require candidates for chiropractic licenses to pass the same basic science examinations as the medical and osteopathic license applicants. In general, chiropractic applicants score rather poorly compared to their medical and osteopathic counterparts.

Chiropractic is more highly regarded in Europe than in America and chiropractic research is more advanced there. Some leading European medical scientists agree that an important spinal factor exists in many functional and pathological conditions. The British Medical Association now recognizes the value of chiropractic in healing. Dr. James Henry Cyriax, a leading British orthopedist, has prescribed or performed manipulation for 40,000 patients

—especially for backaches. He has estimated that 52 per cent of these 40,000 patients have been free of pain after one simple treatment, and nearly all have been eventually cured. According to *Medical World News* of April 2, 1971, Dr. James Mennell of London's St. Thomas Hospital said, "It is indisputable that chiropractic has brought relief to many patients after orthodox treatment has been tried and failed."

In the mid-1970s more than two hundred M.S.s in West Germany formed an organization called *Medical Research and Work Group for Chiropractic.* Dr. Freimat Biectermann, a member of the organization, says, "We medical doctors who have studied and used chiropractic and have proven its indisputable value, cannot understand the negative attitude of medicine toward chiropractic."

Some Americans agree with these European views. Harold T. Hyman, M.D., of the University of Pennsylvania School of Medicine, recently said that "one of the reasons for the popularity of chiropractors is the failure of the medical profession to provide this type of service." W. B. Parsons, M.D., writes in *Applied Therapeutics:* "Those things [chiropractic] are not taught in medical schools. Usually the concept of manipulation is condemned so that new doctors go out in the world with no knowledge, an antipathy toward this most useful method."

Other American physicians attempt to counter such statements by pointing out that many back pains are symptoms of more serious disorders, including coronary thrombosis, duodenal ulcer, cancer of the stomach, and diseases of the uterus, the ovaries, the liver, the kidneys, the prostate, and the intestines.

Most Americans who consult chiropractors today are former patients of medical doctors who were unable to help them. A recent random survey in New York City revealed that 27 per cent of those interviewed had been to a chiropractor and 86 per cent of those who used chiropractic had been helped by it. Sixty-two per cent of this interview group conceded that they had been to physicians without success.

After addressing the pros and cons of chiropractic, I want to summarize the reasons that patients consult chiropractors. First, if a doctor does not possess the knowledge, skill, or inclination to meet the patient's needs, the patient will stop using doctors entirely and look elsewhere for treatment. If you accept the theory that most illnesses are self-limiting and/or psychosomatic in origin, any skillful attention will have an impact and will be given credit for the cure.

Part of the skillful attention a chiropractor offers is his willingness to take time and invest his energy establishing a relationship with each patient. Surveys conducted by health departments indicate that chiropractors, in contrast to physicians, take time to listen, to respond to questions, and to show a personal interest in the patient. Most important, however, is the chiropractor's willingness to touch—"the laying on of hands." The chiropractor's massage releases tension, which modern medical theory strongly suggests is one of the antecedent conditions to all disease.

Since drugs and surgery are not involved, the practice of chiropractic is considered an art. Medicine cannot be all art and no science, but neither can it be science only and deal with human beings dispassionately and completely objectively, without substantial consideration for their foibles, deficiencies, and anxieties. Chiropractic at the least meets these needs.

To conclude my comments on chiropractic, I am amazed that American doctors continue in the late 1970s to be highly defensive about chiropractic, and have not tried to incorporate the best of the chiropractic skills into their medical repertoire.

Dave is a lawyer in his middle thirties. He has the qualities of intellect and precision that you expect from that profession, but the vitality behind his eyes and the way ideas flow from his mind suggest many other dimensions of the man.

He is deeply involved in holistic healing. I will use one of his healing experiences to introduce another brief healing Chautauqua. As an aside, I will simply mention that one of Dave's legal activities in a general practice is helping alternative healers with their legal problems, a fascinating topic in itself, but not germane here.

In 1974, while traveling in Asia, Dave became ill. He was in an isolated rural area of Nepal and found himself so weak that he could barely move. His urine turned black, and, with no medical aid available, Dave feared that he had hepatitis. He rested for several weeks and eventually the symptoms vanished.

Before his trip, Dave had been developing his self-awareness as a natural part of his own personal development. The result of this effort was a heightened sensitivity to his own body and emotional state. Following the experience in Nepal, Dave returned to this country and for the next two years there was a change in the character of his life.

Dave found himself in an uncertain physical state, but was unable to pinpoint the difficulty. In addition, his emotional state was unstable with fairly abrupt swings toward low morale and depressed periods.

Dave's approach to improving his health was holistic. First, he focused on his entire body, and using his own set of meditation exercises in his mind's eye he scanned the nooks, crannies, and organs of his body. There was a suggestion that something was awry in the abdominal area. To check on his own instincts, Dave made three independent moves. He saw a physician, had a psychic reading, and saw an acupuncturist for a pulse diagnosis.

Dave generally had seen physicians only in the case of accidents or major organic dysfunction and for diagnosis. His most common contact with a doctor had been for laboratory testing and diagnosis; frequently another healer had been consulted for managing treatment. In this case the doctor's laboratory tests indicated trouble with the liver, probably stemming from the hepatitis-like incident in Asia.

The psychic reading was done by a medium who specialized in sensing things about the physical body. His reading was specific. He predicted that Dave would have kidney trouble in about two years. Dave took this to mean that his current trouble was probably in the digestive tract.

The acupuncturist's diagnosis was not only specific but immediate. She said half his liver had been destroyed, and, since the liver is considered in acupuncture to be the psychological repository for anger and intense emotion, Dave's emotional gyrations were connected to the liver damage.

Dave decided to receive a series of acupuncture treatments intended to aid the body in its natural repair of its damaged liver.

Dave was still receiving the acupuncture treatments when I talked with him. He commented that on a physical level he was unable to tell if his liver had healed, but his emotional stability had improved substantially, and therefore he was convinced that both his physical and emotional state had improved because of the acupuncture treatments.

Dave experienced an unusual side effect from his acupuncturist's efforts. After she had been treating him for a few weeks, she found it necessary to be out of town for several days. During her absence Dave awoke one morning with a stabiing pain in his right shoulder and was unable to raise his right arm without experiencing severe discomfort. He discovered an inflamed area near his armpit. Later that day a friend who is a pyschic healer looked at Dave's shoulder area and was able to sense an irritation deep in the flesh near the bone. The pain was dealt with quickly and dramatically by the psychic healer. He appeared to go

136

into a trance, and placed his hands on Dave's shoulder. For a moment Dave sensed a hot and tingling sensation in the sore area and then the pain disappeared.

When his acupuncturist returned and heard his tale she exclaimed: "Oh, yes, an emotional reaction like that is common while the liver is being worked on. That shoulder was experiencing anger."

Was the whole affair a psychosomatic aftermath to Dave's Asian illness? He doesn't think so. Dave insists that he has developed his sensitivities to such an extent that he can actually experience small changes or foreign material in his body.

Of all the fringe healing arts, it is most appropriate that we give some special attention to acupuncture—a 5,000-year-old medical technique that made news headlines in the Western world after our ping-pong team visited China in 1971. Since then, hundreds of articles have been written on the subject and a number of books have been published for American readers. Acupuncture is an ancient Chinese system of medicine in which slender needles are placed in a person's skin to a shallow depth in order to cure illness, stop pain, and produce anesthesia. Unfortunately, no one really knows why it works. (Examine some of the books listed in the Chapter Notes if you want to know more about the healing experiences people have had with acupuncture.)

For our purposes it is important to examine the premises underlying the positive value of acupuncture as a healing art. The first is that no bodily intervention is required for diagnosis. No samples of body fluids or tissues are taken. No x rays. No laboratory tests of any kind. No exploratory surgery. Diagnosis is accomplished by examining the patient carefully, asking about *everything* that could influence his or her health, listening to the patient's breathing, and feeling the patient's pulse.

The second major premise of acupuncture is that the

causality of illness, not merely the symptoms, must be treated. The total person is treated, and diagnosis attempts to identify specific causality. The major information source for determining causality of illness are the pulses.

The Chinese believe that the highest level of diagnosis in acupuncture occurs when the healer requires only that the patient be in his presence. Perhaps the patient and the healer sit together for a while. The healer perceives the patient at some unconscious level, intuits the cause of the illness. Every acupuncturist strives to achieve this profound level of interaction with a patient, but most depend on taking the pulses to make a diagnosis.

The pulses are taken by placing the tips of the first three fingers of each hand on the radial artery at about the same place on both wrists that Western doctors use. By using both light and deep touches, twelve different pulses can be discerned. Each of the twelve pulses is related to specific organs of the body, and each pulse has twenty-eight qualities associated with it. Each quality is an indication of a specific illness or disease. Acupuncturists must develop an extreme sensitivity with the fingertips over a long period of training in order to perform pulse diagnosis. Most doctors scoff at the pulse-taking used by acupuncturists. No anatomy book any physician ever studied in medical school even mentions the existence of the pulse configurations used in acupuncture.

The third premise of acupuncture is based on the assumption that all illness comes from interruptions of life-energy flows. The energy flow through the body occurs along a network of lines called meridians. When a pulse diagnosis has been made, the specific illness suggests a set of blockage points along the meridian lines and the needles are inserted at these points. Once the energy-flow balance has been restored, the body can begin to heal itself.

Again, no occidental book on anatomy mentions meridians. There appears to be no obvious physiological evidence of their existence in spite of numerous reports and theories on the subject.

In summary then, acupuncture is itself an holistic healing system that attempts to facilitate healing by restoring and balancing the natural flow of life energy without the use of drugs or surgery. It is impressive and attractive to Westerners who believe in holistic healing. It makes little difference to most people that the way acupuncture works is not understood. Most people I have talked with in preparing this book care most about the end results of a particular healing method but they are selective about the healing system they choose. The choice often depends on the individual and his or her prejudices about a particular healing method. Any number of theories, ideas, and speculations have been made about the effectiveness of acupuncture. For example, many doctors admit that just getting medical attention of any kind will give relief to more than one-third of all patients. Other observers believe that when there is a 5,000-year record of success behind a healing system, the patient is often hypnotized or suggested into getting well—a kind of giant placebo effect.

Other ideas about acupuncture include its short-circuiting the nervous system so the pain signals can't get through; the possibility of a kind of Chinese cupping where the needles reduce inflammation by drawing blood from inflammed areas; and the existence of tiny tubes that actually carry the body's bio-electricity.

What most people forget is that accupuncture is actually an ancient metaphysical method from another culture. If I had been raised in the appropriate physical setting, had acquired the typical attitudes of another culture, and had experienced the conditioning of acupuncture treatments through my entire life, I almost certainly would be writing this section very differently. The same thing could be said, of course, about any healing belief system. How much can flow across cultural or societal barriers? Patients of today are trying to find out.

In working with the body dimension in attempts at holistic healing, a vital factor obviously is the patient's development of body awareness. This takes a myriad of forms. There are the joggers, exercisers, meditators, sensitivity trainees, and many more. Generally, these new activists are in their mid-thirties and upward—when the taken-for-granted youthful body has started producing small pain signals and body sensitivity is developing the hard way. These holistic seekers tend to be in good condition: no excess weight, good body tone, looseness and grace of movement, clear eyes, and a vital demeanor. They don't smoke, drink moderately if at all, and pay careful attention to their diet.

The process of becoming more deeply attuned to changes in your body can be unsettling at first. Receiving a steady flow of messages from the body after years of near silence frequently causes further deep changes in mental attitude and even more focus on physical lifestyle, thus making the process self-perpetuating, and in some cases even obsessive.

The Chinese believe that the best doctors are those who, by working with the pulses, pick up the signals that enable them to prevent disease before it begins. The body-oriented holistic self-healer aspires to the same goal.

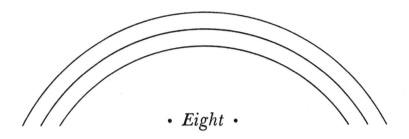

Eight

Healing the Mind

It has been only in this century, and especially since the 1920s, that individual Americans have sought treatment voluntarily for mental conditions that in earlier times they simply would have learned to accept. In the nineteenth century and earlier, only highly disturbed people, presumably psychotics and psychopaths, were attended to openly, and they were committed to penal-like institutions where they had no choice but to accept whatever limited and often misguided treatment forms were available.

In earlier times, when a wealthy person exhibited bizarre behavior he or she was called eccentric. A poor person who behaved in the same way was labeled crazy. Such social phenomena still exist to some extent. Following the impact of Freud's work, however, there has been a shift of national attitudes regarding mental disturbances. We have moved from ignoring or hiding mental problems to seeking help at the drop of a hat and speaking openly in casual social settings about our therapists. Our mental health pendulum has swung so far that we have been accused of indulging in an orgy of mental analysis.

In the last thirty or forty years, as we have learned to accept that mental disturbances are as much a natural part

141

of living as physical malfunctions, there has been an increase in the available mental health resources. The focus of popular psychotherapy has shifted from attempting to cure serious mental disturbances to supporting and counseling people through the everyday problems of life. And recently another shift has occurred; the person who feels stalled in his or her emotional life now finds a plethora of therapists available to help with emotional growth.

By my definitions, the range of mind-healing activities is broad and would include all of the following examples and more: therapy for seriously ill mental patients, whether institutionalized or not; analysis for the person who can never hold a job because of conflicts with other people; counseling for the person who has experienced severe depression since the death of a family member; personal development for the individual who wants to be able to deepen the sense of intimacy in his or her relationships; counseling for the student who has difficulty concentrating and studying; and training in decision-making for the executive who vacillates on important issues. A wide range of mind-oriented concerns, both emotional and cognitive—all of these I view as in the service of healing the mind.

Thomas Kiernan, author of *Shrinks, Etc.: A Consumer's Guide to Psychotherapies,* points out that the same kind of demand effect has occurred in mental health as occurred earlier in physical health. When information about treatments become more widespread, the symptoms of the disorders they were designed to ameliorate rise in the populace also. Much of the additional demand for mental healing comes from a new attitude of unwillingness to live with mental and emotional difficulties. Is the rest psychosomatic? In the matter of physical health there are many examples of communities that experience an increase of medical problems in the population when they are able to get a physician to live in their town, following a long period of living without one.

142

Before going into specific case illustrations as in the last chapter, a general comment: my assumptions here are that *mentally* as well as *physically* it is possible to be born, evolve through a multitude of capabilities, and experience many aspects of life all as a natural progression of living; and whenever the harmonious natural flow that is our birthright is interrupted, whether on the physical or the mental plane, healing can intervene to restore the harmony.

John is a classic case of the boy from a poor family who has been upward bound most of his life. He was born near the time of the stock market crash in 1929, was brought up during the Depression of the 1930s, and was just old enough to serve in the military at the end of World War II. Veteran's benefits financed his college degree—the first one in his family. He served a second time during the Korean War and earned more veteran's benefits, while developing seemingly infinite energy and a limitless desire "to get ahead." Ten years later he had a doctorate and was a respected and reputable professor at a prestigious university. He was married, with two children; owned two cars and a large house.

That situation changed dramatically in the course of three years. John's marriage ended chaotically, and he found himself living in a tiny one-room apartment. He was in poor physical condition as a result of two major accidents. His interest in professional activities had deteriorated to the point where he could barely function in his work.

It is now ten years later that I am interviewing John about his holistic healing experiences. He is a healthy-looking, casual man who appears to be much younger than his nearly fifty years. John has done much experimenting in the last ten years and a totally new lifestyle has evolved for him.

His involvement with holistic healing all began after an

emotional chat with a close professional friend who suggested a visit with a professional therapist. The therapist, in turn, suggested that John join a therapy group. The first group John attended was a weekend workshop that focused on loneliness. The exercises and techniques affected him deeply and initiated a long involvement with groups.

Some of the groups were body-oriented. John learned relaxation exercises, massage, movement and body toning, diet and fasting, Yoga, and more.

In therapeutic groups he was encouraged to share his feelings as he interacted with other members. Gestalt, encounter, psychosynthesis, psychodrama, neo-Reichian, and bioenergetics were some of the therapies he sampled.

In other settings he meditated, chanted, drew pictures, wrote songs, bathed in hot springs, acted, danced, played, and wrestled. Whatever group focus, John found himself with people deeply involved in developing their self-awareness, and then using that self-awareness to improve the quality of all aspects of their life.

When I asked John what were the most important specific things he had learned to do, he smiled and said, "To relax and to breathe."

When I asked John to name the most important experience he'd had, he responded that it was the year that he had worked on a one-to-one basis with a bioenergetic therapist. The insights he gained from that contact have apparently changed his life in profound ways.

The dust jacket of Alexander Lowen's book *Bioenergetics* proclaims: "The revolutionary therapy that uses the language of the body to heal the problems of the mind." Let's see how that holds up.

In contrast to the Freudian-derived therapies that generally offer "talking cures," bioenergetics focuses on nonverbal information taken directly from the body. The basic premise of bioenergetics is that the life of a person is the life of his or her body. Any change in body state influences all other aspects of being, and any change in mind or spirit influences the body. Lowen clearly supports the notion that the several facets of being are highly interdependent.

The therapy emphasizes breathing exercises, moving, feeling, self-expression, and sexuality. Restrictions on these basic functions of life generally are not voluntarily self-imposed but come from the society at large. As I pointed out earlier, we do not live in a culture that emphasizes the importance of physical health. Traditionally, good body condition has often been ignored in favor of the pursuit of power, prestige, and possessions. When a person is in poor physical shape it often affects his or her energy level and capacity for feeling.

What attracted John to bioenergetics was the possibility of returning to the natural attributes of every animal organism—freedom, grace, and beauty. Lowen describes these goals this way: "Freedom is the absence of inner restraint of this flow in movement, while beauty is a manifestation of the inner harmony such a flow engenders. They denote a healthy body and also, therefore, a healthy mind."

There again is the message so many of the alternate healing techniques offer—a return to harmony and naturalness.

The bioenergeticist views the body as an energetic system in constant interaction with the environment. The negative energy of a grouchy person has the potential to pull you down, and a crisp, beautiful sunrise can give you a lift.

A highly "charged" person, one with a high level of personal energy, is thought to be more resistant to negative influences. Special exercises are used to increase the charge.

As a person's energy increases, self-expression opens up, and a stronger sense of feeling returns to the body. Therefore, the emphasis of bioenergetics is always on the specific qualities of breathing, feeling, and movement. From these activities the therapist can obtain information about the current energetic functioning of the individual and try to relate this to his or her life history. The hope is that this two-pronged approach to body and history will slowly reveal inner conflicts. The resolution of any inner conflict will increase a person's energy level.

John told me a fascinating story relating to the process I've just described. When he first started seeing the bioenergetics therapist, the therapist pointed out that John carried his shoulders pulled in to his body and hunched up as though he were perpetually braced against an icy wind.

The therapist showed John how the chest muscle armor that hunched his shoulders also restricted his breathing, especially at times of tension or stress. That same muscle tightness seemed to stiffen his lower jaw and harden the lines of his face.

The therapist proved to John that the muscle armor really existed and showed him what to do to make it disappear. John would lie on a mattress on the floor, and following the therapist's instructions, assume a head-back position and start a deep breathing exercise. When the therapist gave the word, the breathing would be joined by John's legs kicking rhythmically and his fists pounding in unison. Sometimes John would make a sound with each exhalation. With arms and legs churning, and the heavy breathing flooding his system with oxygen, John simply had to "let go," to get involved in making the complex exercise work.

When the exercise ended John experienced a few moments of feeling he was reborn. His face felt wider, fuller, and more alive. His body seemed lighter, softer, and taller. He said that for a minute or two he looked at the world through new eyes, and when he saw himself in the mirror, he appeared changed. His skin color looked healthier and he exuded vitality.

After a few moments, however, the real world flooded

146

back into John's consciousness. As the muscle armor reasserted itself, the energy charge drained away. John claims, however, that he was left with an afterglow to remind him of the new way of being he had briefly experienced.

This exercise was repeated, often in modified forms, many times and John was encouraged to share anything that came into his mind or any sensation he felt while in the softer mood. One or another aspect of his feelings for his mother often came up.

In a review of his history with the therapist, John related that his parents had been divorced when he was an infant and that he had been raised by his grandparents. John had always used the word "abandoned" when he spoke of his mother.

Further bioenergetic exercises followed. John was encouraged to experience all his feelings towards his mother in an attempt to discharge his negative energy toward her.

In a slow, subtle way changes occurred. John started a correspondence with his mother after being out of touch for twenty years. As a result of this renewed relationship with his mother, his references to her became less frequent and not as negative as before. John says that his whole chest area feels more flexible and he proudly displays his shoulders, which have dropped a full two inches.

Most important, he says, anytime his shoulders hunch or his breathing becomes shallow and ragged, he is aware of it. He knows now that for most of his life he was unable to sense the many subtle actions and messages of his body. When John receives these signals now he knows at least that something is happening. Sometimes the cause can be determined; if not, he simply experiences, without resistance, what is happening.

I will let Jason speak for himself by using excerpts from his taped interview to describe his involvement with holistic healing.

Jason is a psychiatrist who is in his early forties. He is in the prime of his professional life. He teaches and does research in a medical school and also maintains a private psychiatric practice.

When I told him what I was doing and showed him the outline of the book, he became animated. Here are some of the things he said to me.

I got interested in holistic medicine at a time when I wasn't very satisfied with my health. I was feeling chronically depressed and had been in psychoanalysis for a while. I had done all the things one does to try to understand what was going on with me.

Finally, about three years ago I decided that my efforts just weren't going anywhere. I was feeling bad; still chronically depressed; my spirits waxed and waned; nothing really felt very good to me.

I was in private practice at the time, and I tried a number of ways to change my health status. I found I could stay on anti-depressant medication and feel fairly good but I could never overcome whatever was bothing me.

Quite by accident, I happend to read an article about meditation in the newspaper and started meditating within a matter of a few months after that.

That's where I began and meditation has been a major factor in my life ever since. I've continued and all those things that were bothering me stopped almost immediately.

Also, I've paid some attention to body work—done some Rolfing, polarity massage, self-healing exercises, bionergetics, and Feldenkrais work. All of these activities have been very effective in helping me feel better about myself.

Finally I began dealing with allergy troubles which have plagued my whole family. Before we moved here from another state we had recurrent bouts of headaches, sore throats, and nausea. We had all kinds of evaluations to try to find out what was happening.

My wife, who was bothered the most, had the usual series of skin tests and some injections were prescribed. These helped. We went through the same process with our son.

When we moved to this state five years ago we had all the allergies in pretty good control with drugs. However, in this new environment the balance fell apart and our allergies returned.

148

We went to a new allergist, got skin tests, and he asked us to wait six months until he knew what our local allergies were going to be. But even when we did all that, it just never helped much.

At that point my young son had a bout with croup which became pneumonia. We tracked that down and it looked like it had an allergic origin. We decided we had to do something!

Quite by accident, my wife, on a bus trip with the local home economics club on the way to visit a cannery, was sitting next to a fine old lady who has written a couple of books on cooking. They started talking and Mrs. Cory said: "Well, you know, you just got to get your diet straight." This suggestion to my wife started a whole new direction in our family's approach to food. We've considered it from an allergy perspective and as a result we avoid certain foods.

We have tended to do this on an elimination diet in order to get free of all symptoms that are identified as food-relating allergy. After we have cut way back, then we add one food at a time until we determine a suitable diet.

The whole family has done it, even though my older children don't always honor their diet in the social world of their friends. But by and large, when they get to feeling poorly they will back off and go on the diet for a week or two. Everybody in the family has a different way of going about this, but all have an increased sense of health maintenance and responsibility.

We have had very good luck. This past year, no one was down with a real cold or flu, only a few light cases. Usually, everybody in the family will have one severe bout a season with these respiratory ailments.

Three of the five of us have learned Transcendental Meditation, but I'm the only regular practitioner. My wife will meditate when there is stress in her life. Say the roof is falling in and the house is on fire. She finds meditation is not a particularly pleasant experience. Instead of quieting the mind, it seems to stir her up and is not pleasant. But, on the other side, she does find the meditation experience physically relaxing. Kind of a curious paradox. My oldest boy has learned to meditate, but has never really done it with any regularity at all.

I can't quite blend the new things I've learned with my own work as a psychiatrist. One part of it has to do with my being somewhat tradition bound in what I do with patients. I'm stuck in my identity role model, tradition, and patient expectations.

Even though I have new ideas of healing I still have a lot to learn. Probably until I can reorganize my own conceptual model, I can't quite get the old and new ideas of healing together.

They are like separate compartments. In my life, in my family's life we do this, but for my patient's life I do that. Part of it really has to do with my still being a rather conforming individual in the sense that it says in the book, right there, that a psychiatrist must do the following things. I think I'm still kind of shy about moving out of that space. It took me a couple of years before I could talk openly about meditating.

I had a patient recently who had a lot of psychosomatic difficulties and would have profited enormously from meditation. It would have allowed him to sit quietly, relax, and mellow out—just what he needed most. But my suggestion wasn't acknowledged and the subject never came up again.

I know a rather traditional analyst who was one of the first people to take *est* [Erhard Seminar Training]. I'm so impressed by the multiplicity of healing opportunities available today. I find I personally use medications much less. I suspect the prescriptions I write for patients reflect this shifting attitude.

It has taken some searching, but while writing this book I was able to speak with several physicians who, like Jason, are starting to break out of the allopathic mold. In my small sample of changing allopathic physicians the majority were psychiatrists, and the most common new healing activity among them was meditation.

Of all the mind-oriented healing activities, why does meditation appear to be the most popular not only for physicians, but people in general?

If I were to be purely analytical in answering that question, I would say that our civilization is at a stage where individuals are vigorously seeking ways to control their physiological reactions to psychological events. We live in a stress-provoking world. The stress stimulus can range from our inner uncertainty all the way to massive world problems. Our technological age is probably testing the human organism's capability of adjusting to disturbing environmental changes more than it has ever been tested.

150

The pace, nature, and quality of our lives may be producing more unsettled stomachs and high blood pressure than we have yet realized.

When we have little self-awareness, minor ailments often go unnoticed and can become the major illnesses of later years. The individual who has developed self-awareness recognizes the body's signals and looks for ways to respond to them immediately.

In our country the most accepted means of stress control have been based on the meditation systems of the Orient. The actual practice of meditation is deceptively simple. Transcendental Meditation (TM), the type most popular in this country, begins with the meditator sitting upright in a comfortable position. You close your eyes and silently repeat to yourself a mantra—usually syllables taken from the Hindu holy books and chosen for the effect of the sound rather than for any meaning. You repeat the sound rhythmically in synchronization with your breathing, and allow any thoughts that appear to drift away and dissipate.

When your mind has become completely quieted, you have "transcended" the consciousness of everyday awareness and presumably can experience another awareness believed to be the source of all creative energy and intelligence.

One reason for the popular success of TM is that it has had a good press. Much has been made of studies done at British and American universities that measured such physiological effects as oxygen consumption, lactate levels in the blood, and brain wave patterns before and during meditation. The data suggest that the nervous system becomes stabilized during meditation and describe the meditator's state as one of alert restfulness, which sounds like a very desirable state to be in.

Research also indicates that the more often you practice TM, the less desire you have for alcohol, tobacco, and hard drugs. Meditators report experiencing higher energy, feel-

151

ing more peaceful and serene, and making subtle changes in their lifestyles. Many practitioners slow the pace of their life, take on fewer new responsibilities, and seem more involved with the responsibilities they already have.

Meditators I've talked with say things like: "My problems don't seem as pressing." "I can sense my body in ways I never believed possible." "I feel more open to people than I ever have in my life." "I enjoy life more than ever."

What none of the reports I have read mention are how many start meditation and simply are not able to do it, or drop out fairly soon. I suspect the numbers would be surprisingly large. One man told me that he was unable to meditate on a regular basis. He complained that he often fell asleep. However, he found meditation invaluable during a crisis period. Through meditation he was able to pull himself back together and deal with the crisis better.

One businessman described meditation as "un-American." He said it causes people to withdraw from the competitive aspects of our culture which are essential to business health and growth. "Horatio Alger would never have been a meditator," he said. On the other hand, another businessman views meditation as merely a practical technique that helps him cope with business pressures.

Harry is like an old friend who lives down the street; the friend to whom you've said "hello" for twenty-five years. He is not intrusive, but gives the sense of being available for contact. I knew that Harry was married, had worked for the telephone company for forty years, and had been retired for over ten years, and was a few weeks shy of being seventy-eight years old. I learned these facts from a mutual friend who suggested that Harry would have some interesting things to say about health. My friend was right.

On a sunny afternoon Harry and I sat and talked in his open woody house at the top of the hill. He was very

152

willing to chat about himself, but preferred that I ask specific questions.

I learned that Harry was born, raised, and schooled in the Midwest in a family deeply involved with fundamentalist Methodist ideas. When he went to college he learned by chance that the nearby Unitarian Church held dances in the basement of its building. That impressed him, and from that day on he has been a Unitarian.

He seemed ill at ease when I mentioned spiritual beliefs. "I'm an organization man," he said. "I've worked hard on administrative tasks for the church for years and I've taken hundreds of their classes, but I don't think of myself as spiritual."

Sports were important to Harry in school, and his memories of those sixty-year-old successes seem fresh in his mind. I suspect that his attitudes towards his body were developed back then, and continue to influence the body awareness he has now.

In recent years Harry has been exploring different ways to maintain his physical health. His efforts are quite amazing to me. A partial list of his body-oriented explorations would include aerobic exercises, breathing exercises, Yoga, stretching, Feldenkrais, self-massage, polarity massage, reflexology, biofeedback, Tai Chi Ch'uan, and nutrition. As Harry tried these body activities over a period of time, he stayed in touch with his family doctor who arranged appropriate laboratory tests to monitor Harry's physical condition. But that was all the doctor did. Harry stoutly avoids all medication. He says he's afraid of the side effects.

From this large mixture of body development and awareness techniques, Harry has carefully selected over a period of time a combination uniquely suited to his needs. As he talked about his body routine, he started demonstrating parts of it. Some is done in bed in the morning after awakening, another part in the bedroom before dressing, and the rest in the kitchen while he prepares breakfast.

153

I watched in fascination the flexibility and agility of this elderly man as he performed a sample of his daily forty-five-minute routine of body-toning.

Harry credits this body work with lowering his blood pressure, ending his early morning backaches, ending the arthritic pains in his back, hip, and knee, and giving him increased energy. He shares his body experiences with his friends in an exercise class he teaches at the local Senior Center.

When I talked to Harry about his emotional life, his eyes turned soft and I sensed him drifting away. He described himself as "a man who has been a little nervous most of my life." He spoke quietly of a previous marriage that ended after twenty years, of two daughters who should have received more of his energy and attention, and of problems with ulcers.

Several years ago, he participated in an encounter group at his church, and another door opened for him. His own insight combined with feedback from the group suggested the need for work with his emotions. In earlier times of crisis he had seen psychiatrists but he felt the exposure had been of limited value.

Through the church group and a therapy group he also joined, Harry has been able to explore several different therapies. Yet, he was candid in admitting that it is not easy for him to share his innermost feelings. Even when he knows he needs the counseling, he still finds the therapeutic interaction threatening.

No one really knows how to match a person to the most suitable therapy. It's mainly a matter of trial and error. Encounter groups were not comfortable for Harry so he sampled Gestalt therapy, bioenergetics, and transactional analysis. For one reason or another he discredited them all. Then he met a Jungian therapist and the match was made. Today he stays in touch with a Jungian therapist whom he sees whenever he senses a need for counseling. Harry told me that if he were ever in trouble he would see a Jungian "because they understand old people better."

My sense of Harry is that with his church, his body work, his counseling resources, and the other aspects of his personal and family life, he is doing well. Harry is not on any old people's shelf. He is a vibrant, warm man whose life process is very much on the move.

Harry's comment about Jungian therapy was so intriguing that I decided to look into it further. Jung was considered the most brilliant of Freud's early associates. He broke with Freud to find a substitute for the heavy emphasis on sexual motivation in Freudian psychotherapy. Jung's replacement therapy was, however, extremely complex.

Jung claimed that people are not driven by sexual instincts, but by the entire set of myths and symbols of the race and culture into which they are born. The inheritance from one's race supersedes and controls the individual's personal unconscious, Jung believed.

Working from this premise, Jung required that an individual retrace his own infancy and the beginning of his own race and culture in order to understand and overcome neurosis. A tall order, even more than Freud asked of his patients.

In Jungian analysis the disharmony within the patient's psyche is resolved through an interaction between the personalities of the patient and the therapist. There are four stages: free association and dream analysis, elucidation, education, and transformation. In the first stage, the therapist seeks uncensored and uninhibited verbal information about the patient's state directly from the patient. Then, in the second stage, the analyst explains the nature of the patient's difficulties. With acceptance of this analysis, the patient can begin to face his or her resistance to change. In the education phase the patient is led toward normal functioning by a specific retraining. In the final stage the patient grows independent of the therapist and returns to normal functioning.

The part of Jungian analysis that Harry liked the most was dream analysis. Because dreams are not taken to be symptomatic in this therapy, their analysis is not threatening to Harry.

Dreams reveal not only the nature and strength of a person's unconscious, but also inform the Jungian therapist about the type and extent of compensation the individual produces as a defense against the weaknesses in his personality. By using a "dream window," the Jungian analyst looks through to an individual's problems, which may appear almost mystical in their origins.

Jung also believed that striving for spiritual significance is the primary individual motivation. If you have sensed some of the complexity of this therapy, you are correct. Thomas Kiernan has pointed out that, "It is by far the most complicated kind of psychotherapy you will undergo."

In reviewing Harry's comments about Jungian analysis, I remember his quiet excitement when he talked about keeping a dream journal, but I suspect a strong friendship and trusting relationship between Harry and his particular therapist may have been more valuable to Harry's mental health than the philosophical details of Jungian analysis.

To conclude this chapter, I want to make several observations about mental healing therapies in general. Earlier, I devoted considerable space to the ability (or lack of it) of the allopathic physician to enhance healing. I have not discussed the corresponding ability of the Freudian psychoanalyst. There are several reasons for this. First, nearly everyone in our society has seen a doctor at some time for some bodily illness or other, but only a few, relatively speaking, have seen a traditional Freudian psychiatrist. Twenty years ago phychiatrists' offices were almost exclusively frequented by well-to-do people. Rarely was a poor person, a drunk, or a drug addict ever analyzed, and the middle class was embarrassed by mental problems. Only in the last two decades have people been willing to use conventional mental health resources openly. As a result there is now a large group of middle-class people who participate in some kind of mental therapy activity. However, most of these people have never actually visited a psychiatrist.

Also, Americans tend to tolerate long, uncomfortable depressions, but go to a doctor for a common cold. Because of this aspect of our culture, most of the holistic healing efforts that this book presents focus more on the body than the mind.

Unlike the dominance of the allopathic physician in healing the body, no single method of psychotherapy holds a monopoly. Even Freudian analysis "would most likely have been nothing more than a footnote in the general cultural and medical history of the Western world" had it not been for the American inclination for self-examination and problem solving, suggests Thomas Kiernan.

Two fascinating results of the proliferation of therapies have appeared in recent studies. The first is that, at the maximum, psychotherapy is 50 per cent effective in resolving mental health difficulties. The second research is that a large percentage of emotional problems are self-resolving, usually within two years. This doesn't produce much of a batting average for psychotherapy, but we must keep in mind that we are discussing an infant science.

Average lay persons cannot differentiate between the many therapies available, and even if they could there is no way to know without trial which approach would be best. It is a bromide among therapists that some people will profit from any therapy, some will not respond to any therapy, and the rest will be helped only by being exposed to the one appropriate therapy. This is an interesting idea, but unfortunately no one knows how to identify the members of each group.

Body healing and emotional healing have at least one important characteristic in common. In the majority of cases a placebo effect is operating, and when a cure is achieved, the treatment that was used at the particular time will be given credit for the cure.

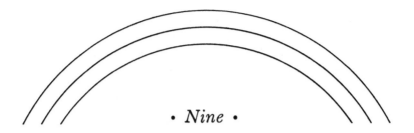

Nine

Healing the Spirit

The word *spirit* has many different connotations and shades of meaning. The dictionary phrase that comes closest to the scope of this chapter is: "An animating or vital principle held to give life to physical organisms."

When I talked to people about their spiritual evolution, they would often mention the word *soul.* Returning to the dictionary to check *soul,* I found such definitions as, "A person's total self"; "Man's moral and emotional nature"; "The immaterial essence of an individual life."

Each of the persons I have interviewed will give their own definitions of spirituality in their separate narratives. The nature of spirituality as a topic requires also that I begin the chapter with a healing Chautauqua. This is to prepare the way for following a delicate, but distinct thread that is common to the narratives that follow.

When I asked individuals where their involvement with holistic healing began, the most frequent answer was emotional troubles. A foundering marriage, interpersonal difficulties at work, child-rearing trauma, or an overwhelming sense of being alone were the kind of events and feelings

159

that started these people on self-exploration paths that led to holistic healing.

Self-awareness and emotional stability achieved by one means or another was invariably followed by a deep concern about the body. So, then, a common experiential healing sequence for many people is in the order of mind, emotions, body and spirit. The commonality of experience ends there, however. The actual division of individuals' healing energy among these human dimensions varies enormously from person to person.

The idea that each of us is born whole and healthy in mind, body, and spirit was emphasized by many people I interviewed. Some allowed for the reality of birth defects, but most people believed that poor health was a direct result of the accumulation of toxic living experiences. This is a marvelous viewpoint. It suggests the possibility of returning to the wholeness that is our birthright by healing the effects of living in today's stressful world.

It is common enough to talk about being physically ill and emotionally ill, but what does it mean to be spiritually ill? Peter Ford, a psychiatrist who participated as a physician in a chaplaincy training program at a hospital for many years, defines spiritual illness in this way: "Spiritual illness may be defined as an emotional and cognitive malady that arises out of the human failure to respond to God's love. It results in a three-way separation: a separation of the individual from God, from himself, and from others."

Ford goes on to write about the degree of separation, the period of love-deprivation, and the relationship between these factors and an individual's happiness and ability to function adequately in his or her environment.

I find Ford's ideas appealing because his language allows us to discuss spiritual illness in a specific way. If the God he speaks of can be taken broadly to mean "a higher power," then you will discern ties between Ford's clinical viewpoint and the interviews in this chapter.

160

What are the clinical signs and symptoms of spiritual illness? To answer this question I must deal with an immediate potential confusion. The manifestations of both spiritual and psychological illness are similar. The difference between a depression caused by a lack of love in a person's interpersonal life is not easily differentiated from a depression which comes from a spiritual problem. This should come as no surprise. We have seen that it is extremely difficult to separate emotional from organic conditions in other types of healing. When a patient complains of repeated chest pains that extend to the left shoulder and down the left arm, it is difficult for a physician to determine whether the patient is suffering from coronary artery disease or "cardiac neurosis," which can mimic coronary artery disease in nearly every detail. The neurotic condition is caused by tension and fatigue, however, and generally has a much brighter prognosis.

Some symptoms of spiritual illness are a sense of hopelessness and despair, extreme loneliness, feelings of guilt, fear of death, and the sense of being unloved and unwanted. Clearly, with any of these symptoms, the zest for living is gone. In serious cases, suicidal thoughts and attempts are common.

Peter Ford proposes that rejection is the primary cause of spiritual illness. Rejection of self and rejection by others is part of his thesis, but rejection of God is the dominant cause. We are treading on delicate theoretical ground now, but I offer Ford's thoughts as among the most impressive I have discovered. The practical point is that Ford can construct a therapeutic approach and attempt to help patients diagnosed as spiritually ill because he has a working principle.

I have found in my interviews and studies that there is a great deal of uncertainty and ignorance concerning the spiritual dimension of life. Too often spiritual health is thought to be related to an intellectual understanding of formal theology or going to houses of worship regularly.

161

There is also a belief common to Americans that spiritual matters are intuitive and private and that education and rational understanding are inappropriate to them. Moreover, spiritual health issues seem to be treated today with the same uncertainty and secrecy as mental health matters were a few decades ago. Persons who sense spiritual problems are frequently unaware of the resources that they might tap and are unwilling to discuss their problems openly.

The traditional educational pipelines of the churches are bureaucratic and are plagued by all the usual problems of any highly organized institution. Take, for example, the predicament of the minister, rabbi, or priest. He is expected to be administrator, fund-raiser, counselor, spiritual inspiration, and teacher of often recalcitrant and indifferent parishioners. In addition, he is expected to change the parishioners' lives through the single medium of a weekly sermon that is stimulating, inoffensive, witty, profound, biblical in origin, and with minimal contemporary applications so as not to disturb the minds of the more generous supporters of the church's operational budget. As if that weren't enough, the spiritual leader must also relate equally well to persons ranging in age from eight to eighty, with varied educational backgrounds and interests.

Consider some of the other spiritual resources. Apart from bureaucratic and highly organized churches and synagogues, there are the smaller religious movements such as the Church of Christ, Scientist, Scientology, and Jehovah's Witnesses. Beyond that group lie the more obscure religious sects, including the Eastern religions that are now so popular with younger people. Our spiritual resources offer a multitude of confusing options.

It is inappropriate here to develop the case for the failure of churches to meet the spiritual needs of a great many people, but the interested reader is invited to browse in the references in the Chapter Notes at the end of the book.

162

Given that spiritual illness exists and that most people find limited spiritual healing resources to invoke, Peter Ford suggests a means by which spiritual healing can be facilitated. The healing process includes an analytical phase, which determines the nature and extent of the spiritual illness, and a therapeutic phase to deal with the spiritual malady.

When you see Dr. Ford for counseling, he begins by using psychological techniques to determine how alienated from others you are. That requires examining the limits and contents of your environment, your value system, and finally your goals and understanding of the meaning and purpose of life.

Here are some questions that might be asked: How interested are you in community, state, and national affairs? What are your relationships to your spouse, parents, children, employers, and peers? How do you feel about the moral and legal restraints that society places on you? Do you accept yourself, or would you rather be someone else? Whom do you wish most to impress, your family, your friends, or yourself? How important to you are professional success, social recognition, and devotion to family?

Next, an indirect approach is used to learn about the extent of the human-divine relationship in your life. Not considered as meaningful yardsticks are church attendance, the ability to recite large quantities of scripture, or the willingness to pray in public. If, after questioning, it emerges that an individual can only verbalize about God, and there is little or no evidence of love and compassion for others but only self-pity and anger, the human-divine relationship is taken to be very weak.

In the last stage of spiritual analysis there is an attempt to match a person's potential for fulfillment against his actual spiritual condition. Allowances are made for factors such as age, environmental conditions, ethnic background, and religious and social heritage.

The therapy that follows the spiritual analysis involves two ideas: replacement and movement. Replacement means acquiring fulfilling attributes instead of debilitating ones. The therapy tries to exchange hostility for comfort, boredom for purpose, sorrow for joy, inner turmoil for peace, loneliness for companionship, and despair for hope. These are wonderful concepts, but it is a tall order.

In the second (or movement) part of the therapy, the patient is helped to diminish his or her three-way alienation from God, self, and others. The hope is that the therapist who serves as a counselor, educator, and friend can also be a channel through which the love of God can be transmitted.

Ford's approach to spiritual illness is intellectual and practical. The therapy represents a spiritual health resource that offers a secular path to a better state of being to pragmatic, nonreligious people. I've provided only a cursory look at Ford's approach. His book *The Healing Trinity,* offers far more detail to the interested reader.

Ford's work has been influenced by the theologian Paul Tillich, whose key notion was that faith in a higher power must precede belief in that power. This is an essential part of Ford's therapy. Tillich had this to say about prayer:

> Every serious prayer contains power, not because of the intensity of desire expressed in it, but because of the faith the person has in God's directing activity—a faith which transforms the existential stituation.

In the interviews that follow, mention of the power of prayer will occur frequently, and the connection of prayer to healing will be apparent. Yet prayer is mysterious. Is it auto-suggestion, a frame of mind, or a learned technique?

Let me close my discussion of Ford's spiritual therapy with the words he uses when he outlines to a patient his full course of therapy:

When you first come to me, I will love and accept you. When you begin to feel secure in my love, then you must go out and love someone who will respond to your love, and then return to me in order that you might receive more of my love. Next you must go out and love someone who will welcome you, but who will not know how to receive your love, and then return again to me and I will love you. Finally, you must go out and love someone who needs your love, but who will be unwilling to accept it. When you can do this, and remain strong, you will no longer need to return to me, for you will have been healed.

The spiritual path of my friend Beth began very early in her life and continues evolving today. She is an attractive, mature woman in her late thirties. When we talked about healing and spiritual matters we sat in her sunny backyard. Her manner was warm and forthright as she talked to me, giving me the impression that for those moments our conversation was the most important event in her life.

Beth comes from the Bible Belt, a part of our country that is known for ardent religious fundamentalism. In her Lutheran family the adults went to church occasionally, but the children were never allowed to miss.

Beth's family was very concerned about "the right or wrong of things." She was required to pray before bed and she recalls that church was "a drag." Nevertheless, the righteous fervor had an impact on young Beth. How could it have been otherwise? She recalls that when she was eight years old, her mother went to visit relatives and Beth requested a Bible as a returning gift from her mother. Beth still has that Bible.

At fourteen, after her confirmation in the church, she went to Bible camp where she met a pastor she described as "the first person I had ever met who was truly in the spirit." In a highly emotional interaction with this minister, she decided to accept Jesus as her savior. Beth's conversion and open acceptance of Christianity were a turning point that came up often in our conversation.

Through high school she did what was expected of her and lived a moral life—no smoking, dancing, drinking, sex, and on and on. All her friends lived the same way, but as high school ended, Beth's interest in spiritual matters waned. The rightness and wrongness shoes began to pinch.

Leaving home after high school also meant leaving the overt religious life behind. After taking philosophy courses in college, Beth called herself an agnostic, and even tended toward atheism. She realized that she had been "defined and confined" by the religious intensity of her family and leaving home was an opportunity to break out. A word that kept recurring in our chat was rebellion.

After college Beth went on to graduate school and then married at twenty-five. Seemingly overnight she was a wife and mother with a family of her own. Beth has always been a highly energetic woman. Her master's degree in mathematics landed her a laboratory job that became part-time whenever pressures at home demanded more of her time. She is a superb violinist and spent as much time as possible with the local symphony orchestra. And as if all this were not enough, her hobby was working on the political campaigns of candidates she supported.

Somehow, in the midst of all this activity, her family grew to three children and her husband Bill, a very successful businessman, raced alongside her in a similar lifestyle. Then the first signs of trouble appeared. The story is a familiar one. Both Beth and Bill started being sick too much. Just little things. Colds and coughs and such.

Next it was depressions for Beth and an ulcer for her husband. Then problems in their relationship. Except for the obvious physical symptoms, it was as though a secret agent was undermining her entire life. The zest was vanishing.

Beth, with the support and participation of her husband and children, started to look for answers to questions she could not even ask yet. And she did it in her high-energy,

166

"head-lowered-and-charge" manner. She talked to friends and counselors of many kinds. Her entreaty was always the same. "Things are not right, and I want to find out why and do something about it."

That was nine years ago. Many changes have occurred since then. Old activities have fallen away from Beth's life and new ones have taken their place. There were few guideposts along the way. Beth's intense desire to find the root of the problem, coupled with her own intuition, found the path to spiritual healing. The pain of uncertainty was replaced by the chaos of change. Friendships were allowed to wither, money became a constant hassle, and difficult choices were made again and again.

The story of Beth's family and their healing experiences is long and complex. From it, I have tried to extract the thread that best captures Beth's individuality and her method of spiritual healing.

Beth decided to work on a problem that had plagued her all her life—not being able to show her anger or express any very negative feelings. As long as she could remember she had swallowed her anger until it poisoned her. Because of a friend's knowledge and enthusiasm Beth was able to spend one evening a week for nine months in a room where she shrieked at strangers. She was playing Synanon games, a group activity that emphasizes aggressive, hostile interactions as a personal learning device. She learned how to get her anger outside herself instead of letting it fester, and she felt relief from the experience. But she got more than that from Synanon. The incessant hostility of the games tapped levels of her being of which she had never been aware. Not just the deeply buried anger, but her penchant for defending, explaining, and generalizing. And sorrow over her lost dreams of youth. Synanon gave Beth a new way of seeing herself, and after that learning was accomplished she moved on.

After Synanon, Beth sampled many different therapy groups and developed a deep interest in Gestalt therapy.

167

Beth becomes excited when she talks about those days. Everyone in her family participated in the search for self-awareness. For herself, she spoke of having an illusion of having many choices and being "with it."

In the Gestalt group exercises, Beth's alienation from her parents came up frequently and became the core of her efforts in the group. At first she felt strange as she talked to the empty chairs where her father and mother were supposed to be sitting, but she became accustomed to it and her efforts in therapy cleared away old concerns.

Beth learned another valuable lesson—that when she had a problem she should examine her own attitudes first. This awareness from the Gestalt experience led to a new era of improved relations with her parents. Visits became more frequent and satisfying.

Beth and her family experienced a fast-moving period of evolution because of the exposure to Gestalt therapy. There were clothing, lifestyle, grooming, and behavior changes. The children thrived on the candid expression of feelings and the family had never seemed in better physical condition.

By experimentation and questioning, Beth became involved in the practice of Yoga. The difficult Yoga positions left her body aching and uncomfortable, so she developed her own set of body-toning exercises that take only ten minutes a day. Each exercise was selected because it seemed to fit her particular body needs. To improve her body condition further, she took a series of structural integration sessions (Rolfing).

Apparently Beth's development along emotional and body conditioning lines led her back to spirituality. She puts it this way: "There was no special event or external guidance that occurred. I seemed to be tuned into a spiritual vibration. I began to realize that the conversion experience I'd had at fourteen was real."

A number of new experiences followed swiftly. Beth entered a Pecci-Hoffman training period to explore the tie

168

between her emotions and spirit. She went to spiritual communities and met many spiritual leaders. She attended meditation retreats held by a swami from India and her visits with him left her very peaceful.

I was amazed by the efforts Beth had put forth to develop her body, emotions, and spirit; and of course, the process is not complete. For nearly a decade she has involved her family, her energy, and all of her resources to seek a better way of being in this world. She has openly revealed her weaknesses, made difficult choices, changed, and tested her sensitivities again and again.

At the moment, Beth is searching for a spiritual teacher who can help her to feel closer to Christ. This might be through a conventional Christian church but she is not sure. It surely will be a life-long process.

Spending time with Beth was very satisfying for me. She exudes a positive sense of well-being. The most important moment in our conversation came when I asked Beth if she could put into words what the impact of all her efforts were on her everyday life. She replied:

> The work on my emotions seemed to wipe my slate clean and now my spirituality is painting a beautiful picture there. My spiritual path allows me to cultivate my beauty, my love and purity, my innocence, and my surrender. I rely on grace now and I'm able to see beauty in everyone and everything. I'm free from worry and ego attachments. I have more to offer my family than ever before.

Because it figured in most conversations I had with the persons I describe in this chapter, I want to pause for a brief look at the contemporary relationship between healing and Christianity. A review of the historical literature will show that Christianity has carried with it an appreciation of emotional and spiritual factors that influence human life and contribute to healing.

Today it is clear that our health depends to a great extent on emotional factors and therefore ultimately on elements that may not be simply the creation of either our

169

own psyche or the physical world. We appear to be experiencing non-physical forces that affect the health of all people. Here again, the impact of Jungian analysis is felt. Jung and his followers have argued that human beings have a purposeful center of reality. For many people this center is religion and a belief in God. People seldom stay well mentally and physically without finding some way to relate their lives to their center of being. Jung further claimed that the fact that healings do occur to persons who are in spiritual states is evidence that a relation to God is possible and needed.

If a church wants to have a healing ministry and to be a setting for holistic healing, it must practice a theology in which the spiritual power has the gift of healing. In a church with a healing ministry both clergy and laity provide the emotional and spiritual climate in which emotional and spiritual healing can occur. The church can provide a loving community to facilitate healing. Unfortunately, this quality is not often found in a traditional church. People who claim soul-shattering healing experiences are often avoided and looked upon as strange.

Now that we have reviewed the conditions that are necessary for the encouragement of healing within a Christian church setting we can progress by contrast with the experience of the next interview subject, Ann, who has created similar conditions outside of a Christian environment.

Ann and I talked in the living room of her home on a warm summer evening. She is a small woman with a gentle, direct gaze. Ann's presence seems to create a special atmosphere. I think her words will give you a sense of her special qualities. She is a Gestalt therapist, and she begins with a mention of her own therapy groups.

Whenever I do one of my Gestalt training groups, I begin by acknowledging my teachers. I have been doing this for a couple of years, and it occurred spontaneously the first time. Suddenly I

170

found myself acknowledging my mother, and I realized that my mother was my first teacher. Next came Fritz Perls and some of my other Gestalt teachers. Then I offer appreciation for years of sitting zazen (meditation), because I believe it has given me clarity and serenity. I also acknowledge my work in psychosynthesis and my spiritual teacher. All of these people and things have influenced my life and my work.

I have no structured religious background, but I know that in my heart I've always had a sense of spirit. My family is Jewish, but as a youngster I took myself off to Sunday school and sang in the choir of various churches. In college I followed the typical path of declaring myself an atheist.

The big revolution in my life came many years later when I spent a week at Esalen Institute in California. That experience literally flipped my consciousness, and I've never been the same since.

All the people I normally account to were not with me—no husband, no children, no parents. I was able to shed, at least briefly, all responsibilities and the roles I played. When I went to that workshop I was so ripe and ready for the experiences I had.

If you had been able to peek in on my workshop that week you might have wondered what the big deal was. I was in an encounter group and from the outside it would have seemed that we spent an inordinate amount of time just sitting and chatting. We were a very mixed group of people—old and young, fat and thin, attractive and ugly. The kind of people you might collect in a very large butterfly net snapped over a busy sidewalk intersection in any city.

What made the difference, however, was that in that beautiful setting, under the guidance of the group leader, I began to see and appreciate those human beings. It was as though we had left society with its crippling alienation behind. I felt very free and simultaneously very close to those people I had known only a few days.

In that week I grew up from feeling like a little girl to feeling like a woman. I shed so many trappings in my life, both external and internal. I felt an incredible freedom to be myself, and it manifested in all kinds of ways. I took off my glasses that I'd worn all my life; I let my hair down; I took my shoes off; and I took my bra off. I just plain let go.

For the first time in my life I turned my awareness inside to myself. I experienced the beginning of the realization of how the sense of the spirit could permeate my life if I were just open to

171

seeing it and listening to the signs of it in my life. I think it all happened because of love for and from those strangers.

When I returned home, everyone could see that I had changed. At first, some of the changes lasted only a few weeks. I found myself becoming a better listener, able to relax more. As I did more group work, I seemed to be more in tune with my family and friends. Sometimes I knew what they were going to say before they spoke.

Then I started in Gestalt therapy and the road was up and down. At another Esalen workshop I was in deep despair. I began doing meditation about that time. Meditation was and is especially important to me. When I meditate I am totally grounded in the here and now. I love it.

Since that first experience in 1968 it's been continual growth, strengthening and learning more about myself. Especially in the past two years I've sensed a deepening of the spiritual values in my life. I feel freer to move quickly toward and love the people in my group. I've no doubts at all that my open and unabashed willingness to accept and love helps the people with their work in my therapy groups.

Ann told me the story of an illness she experienced that marked another turning point in her life. Each part of a complex problem was solved by applying one element of holistic healing. As I listened to her it was clear that she found the inspiration for putting the pieces together by surrendering herself to spiritual guidance.

About five years ago I was very ill. I was barely able to breathe for a couple of weeks because of an asthmatic attack. I awoke every night about 2:00 or 3:00 a.m. just gasping to catch my breath and filled with fears—how am I going to support my children—how will I be able to work again;—I'll be an invalid.

As the fear choked me, I prayed continuously, saying: "I am the light, I am the Christ light." When I stopped praying the fears rushed in again.

After a couple of weeks of this struggle, one night I prayed for several hours and finally said, "O.K., God, this is it, I can't do this anymore."

I asked for help because I wasn't willing to go to a doctor and be given cortisone for my asthma. I knew intuitively that I shouldn't use drugs. As I prayed, a person's name came through to my

172

consciousness. It was the name of a man I'd known years before. He's a physician turned Reichian therapist and I called him immediately. He gave me the name of the acupuncturist I now see. The first acupuncture treatment gave me almost instant relief from the asthma and the symptoms never returned that badly again.

I realized that things were happening in my body that had begun almost at birth. Several organs weren't working properly. I've continued acupuncture treatments and most of these problems have been dealt with. My physical body has steadily strengthened since that frightening experience.

I know I pray practically all the time. I've found that more and more I can move away from the actual process of my life and invoke spiritual help.

Four years ago, with my family grown and gone and my own inner life richer than it had ever been, I searched for an insight about what to do next. The knowing came to me during prayer. I decided to use Gestalt therapy, as a base for a new life for me and a way of helping other people.

The training period to become a Gestalt therapist was a bittersweet learning time for me. Now, though, I feel truly connected to the community around me. I take some of my identity from this service role, and I like having it.

The work that is happening in my groups is phenomenal, and it's not my work. It's not personally me. The prayer that I use often is: "Let me stand aside so that your energy can be made manifest." In that way, every person in the group can experience his or her divine self. It's really awesome to witness.

I've continued meditation and Yoga and they have helped me become more conscious and aware.

I constantly see evidence all around me of the spirit made manifest. Little things. I walk down the street and there is beauty everywhere. The natural way everything fits together never fails to amaze me.

I've found that when I stop fighting and arranging, everything works out. The right people come along and the right circumstances make themselves available. All I have to do is to release personal control and surrender to a greater power.

I learned that if I don't push and think I must do everything when I set up one of my workshops, everything falls into place—the right people, the right location, and the right conditions.

The most important part is that I have the intention to do it. As I get clearer and clearer about my intention—such as deciding to have fourteen people for a workshop, where we will meet, and that kind of detail—it all comes together. Whenever I am not totally clear about my intentions, whatever I'm trying to do simply does not work out. It's such a beautiful lesson in clarity and surrender.

I continuously acknowledge the power of the spirit. As I walk along and see something beautiful, I'm filled with gratitude. There is so much that's beautiful in my life, and I want to acknowledge it.

I don't feel any connection to formal religion. I read books on the life of Jesus, and I marvel at the beauty of the man. Many people from the church are attracted to the work I do. Both Jesuits and nuns are in my Gestalt groups. I love having them because they are such wonderful, sensitive people.

As my last case subject in this chapter on spirituality, I want to introduce Phil. Though only thirty-five years old, he is prematurely gray. At a distance his gray hair and beard make him appear much older. His voice is resonant with a slight European accent and he speaks in a measured, somewhat formal way. His eyes and body movements, however, are boyish. Although he is physically a small man, something about his presence and demeanor makes him seem much larger.

Our conversation regarding Phil's spiritual healing was very emotional. He told me of events that had occurred so recently that talking about them was almost like living the experience. Phil is the son of a fundamentalist Christian minister and he grew up in a small European country. Religious activities permeated his family's life. There were daily Bible readings and prayers and frequent visits to the church.

When Phil was nine years old, his parents were "saved." In the lexicon of their church that meant an even deeper religious commitment—a total dedication of their life to Jesus and complete devotion to their particular kind of fundamentalist Christianity. That event was to have enormous impact on Phil's life. Two months later, he was taken to a revival meeting knowing that his parents expected him to be saved, too. Phil described the episode this way:

So, of course, according to my parent's schedule I was *saved* along with my brother who is a year older. I felt very uncomfortable during the ceremony. I was awkward, anxious, uncertain, and had a horrible feeling in the pit of my stomach. I stood there embarassed and trembling and muttered something about being saved and giving my life to Jesus. A moment later, I sat down with relief flooding over me. After reflection, I realized that I believed something had happened to me, and I actually had been saved.

Looking back, Phil believes that he was simply trying to do something to please his parents, especially his father, who was a key figure in his life.

My father, as a minister, was a symbol of God for me much more than he was a true father. He was not available to me—rarely around and very stingy with his energy. The only way he could relate to me, or anybody else, was as the minister. I can recall clearly sitting in the pews of his church as a boy. A special little door at the side of the alter would be flung open, and he strode in majestically in his long, black cassock. He seemed strong, God-like, and unreachable.

The intensity of religious fervor increased in Phil's home after the family had been saved. That time was the gestation period for a decision Phil made when he was thirteen. After a gradual buildup of pressure, he totally rejected his religion. He says that dominant negative feelings towards his parents were the reasons. He thought his mother hypocritical and his father unresponsive. He continued behaving, however, in the same way as before, and told his secret to no one.

Not having anything to believe in was terrifying. I lived in abject fear of death, since heaven didn't exist for me anymore. I didn't believe in any kind of purpose to the universe. There was no alternative to my notion that existence was useless and senseless.

Phil lived the next twenty-two years of his life under the influence of a deep fear of annihiliation.

To avoid destruction, I became a glutton for physical experiences —food, wine, sex, travel, mountain-climbing—all the "things" I've been involved with.

As Phil's story approached his recent past, he described a familiar pattern. Stress appeared everywhere in his life. His marriage failed. His work as an engineer became unsatisfying and he changed jobs frequently. He had lived a life of consumption, performance, and achievement and the pressure was getting him down.

The turning point came for Phil as a result of an experience with his six-year-old son Leon. Phil's random visits with Leon were mini-parties with a flood of gifts. The flood became a deluge as Phil began to fear that Leon wasn't all that interested in his visits.

Finally, one day on the telephone, Leon said: "Will you take me somewhere—just the two of us? Let's go to the creek and you don't have to bring me anything."

Imagine the scene. A man and his son strolling along a creek bank in the country. Sunlight sparkling on the water; leaves rustling in the breeze. The breathless chatter of a young boy and the deeper slow murmurs in reply.

There is no startling dramatic climax for this scene. Phil suddenly simply knew everything. He clearly felt his own emptiness and his alienation from the rest of the world. He knew he was a shadow of a man. He told me: "I realized I was living a life of complex coping and I decided that afternoon with Leon to do something about it."

Phil rearranged his life, and made his time, energy, and resources available to start his healing. He learned about therapy groups from a friend and his group experiences were the beginning of a wide range of healing activities. All this happened two years before I talked with him.

About six months ago he found a psychiatrist who led therapy groups aimed at spiritual development. In his group sessions, there was a gradual introduction of spiritual values. Some of the emotional problems of the partici-

176

pants were described as "a fall from grace." The word, God, was mentioned frequently, and the state of being toward which the group members aspired was described as "attributes of God that can exist in us." An important spiritual juncture was coming and Phil's own words describe it best:

I began to suspect that the totally random universe was not so random. Especially in my meditations I began to sense an outer power and harmony which permeates the universe and of which we are a part. After being in the group about three months, one day we were instructed to do an exercise that involved a moving meditation, heavy physical exercise, special breathing techniques, and prayer. We had carefully prepared for this day and I felt open to whatever might happen.

Concentrating on my breathing and carrying a heavy rock representing all the bad things from my past, I trudged up a steep hill. Breathing carefully, I allowed myself through prayer to surrender to the idea that God would take the rock from me. The entire experience moved me so much that I burst into tears and sobbed for a long time.

I knew there was a void in me, caused by my boyhood rejection of religion, which had left me empty, desperate, and lost. The fence around the hole in me had been broken down. The group leader told me: "God has been stalking you all these days."

That night after leaving the group Phil rushed to his ex-wife's home and hugged the confused woman as he blurted out a nearly incoherent promise to be always available to help. After hugging and kissing a sleepy Leon, Phil went to the telephone and woke up his parents three thousand miles away. He told them he loved them, and they made plans for a visit in a few weeks. The next morning he made the first move toward doing what he had always wanted to do—teach. Phil says he feels so much more clear about his life now.

It's as though my psyche and soul have been cleansed. Anything that happens in my life is spiritual. Walking on the street, being in the mountains, looking at the sky, and hugging my son are spiritual.

177

True spirituality is the being of my life—being whole, healthy, and loving. My moral code is that I am responsible for everything in my life—to myself and to God.

Are Beth, Ann, and Phil merely ordinary middle-class neurotics fighting their way through rather predictable life crises? I think not. Their crises were brought on by common toxic living experiences that left them spiritually wounded. However, the ways in which they dealt with their injuries were extraordinary in relation to the general populace. Yet they are typical of the growing breed of holistic health seekers. They sensed their problems and then took all the time and energy that were required to deal with them. Just as a person who suffers physical injury in an automobile accident might become dedicated to physical therapy, Beth, Ann, and Phil have devoted a part of their lives to spiritual therapy. Their spiritual healing was blended with healing the body and emotions and the outcome was holistic healing.

No one has more aptly described the joy that comes with successful spiritual healing than Sam Keen in *To A Dancing God.* He says: "The haze in the air evaporates and the world comes into focus; seeking gives way to finding; anxiety to satisfaction. Nothing is changed and everything is changed. Human existence ceases to be a problem to be solved and becomes a mystery to be enjoyed."

178

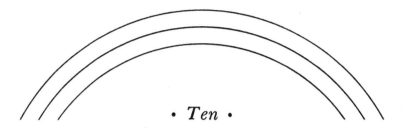

Ten

Self-Healing

In the 1960s and 1970s the nonfiction book market has been dominated by "how-to" books. You can find a how-to book on everything from grooming your armadillo to tuning your zither. With this flood of information has come a steady current of self-help health books covering subjects such as how to take your own blood pressure and what it means or how to palpate (examine by touch) your own body. *The Well Body Book* (1973) by Mike Samuels and Hal Bennett is now a near classic example.

Such books emphasize the learning of a host of largely mechanical medical tasks. Generally their point is that many things that are done infrequently and expensively by doctors and nurses can be done regularly and expertly by people at home. Money may be saved, of course, but more important, people who do these things report a sense of involvement with their bodies in ways they have never before experienced. Even the simple daily ritual of checking your weight variations and relating the changes to what's happening in your life offers an entirely different way of perceiving yourself.

In a rather limited way, self-monitoring activities can be called self-healing in the preventive sense. It is as if we are giving ourselves a continuous physical examination. If we take charge of our own bodies, many illnesses can be detected before they develop into something more complex. The body generally gives many warning messages well in advance of trouble.

The limited self-healing I have just described, though valuable, is not the primary focus of this chapter. Here I am concentrating on healing as a *repair* process that occurs naturally when conditions are right. We seek healers to help us establish the appropriate conditions so the body, mind, or spirit can heal itself, or we become healers of ourselves and help to provide suitable environments for natural healing to take place.

On the first level, we seek out and put together an appropriate combination of healers by evaluating them according to our perceptions and our awareness of what we need. Further, we can monitor their treatments carefully and make adjustments according to our informed sense of what is happening. This kind of self-healing means taking an active, responsible, and managerial approach to staying well, and many of the holistic-healing people I've talked with do just that.

A second level of self-healing is reached when you are, in fact, your own sole healer; when, out of self-knowledge, determination, and will, you gather and focus your own natural energy and possibly seek outside healing energy to facilitate healing. Instead of trying to describe this, I'll let Ann tell you what it's actually like to do it. You will recall Ann as the Gestalt therapist who described her spiritual evolution in Chapter 9.

About two years ago at an out-of-town workshop I was leading, I felt terrible. A migraine headache had my head in a vise and the rest of my body on a torture rack. And as if that weren't enough, I had a painful irritation from the recurrence of an old eye injury. I can't tell you how I knew this, but I sensed the pain was there for a special reason.

About an hour before the workshop was to begin I was in

excruciating pain and I began to pray. My prayer seemed to pull me together and concern about the workshop and other people melted away. There was nothing in this world but me and my pain. I had the insight that the pain was a teacher and a blessing for me. I don't know how I did it, but somehow my shift to a positive attitude allowed me to surrender to the pain. I felt myself enter the core of the pain and stay there while praying. I was totally alone in that place with my pain.

An hour later, when I met the group, the discomfort was nearly gone. I was absolutely amazed. More and more now I find I can enter any pain, become one with it, and accept the pain as a way of closing everything else out and allowing me to turn inward. After I do this, the pain eases very quickly. Before I was able to do this, a migraine headache would build to a shattering peak, then slowly taper off, and all this could take from several hours to several days.

Prayer is powerful. It's like going inside and recontacting my divine self. When I want to do something like relieve pain or heal myself I create images in my head of what I want to happen. The stronger and clearer my intentions become, the closer what actually happens comes to my images. If I sense some part of my body in distress, I image it as a whole and healthy pain. I bathe the pained part in healing energy which I visualize as white light.

After my first experience with entering the pain of a migraine headache, I started envisioning the veins in my head and the pressure build-up around them creating the headache. Then, in my mind's eye, I bathe that part of my head in white light to relieve the pressure, and it works.

I've learned that in order to heal myself I must not resist the illness. Instead I surrender and go into it; I turn off all thoughts; I experience the illness totally at that moment. After I've done that, I visualize the affected area and bathe it in healing energy. The whole process is like a meditation. All of my personal energy is focused on myself at that moment.

One of my favorite images when I pray is being held in God's hand or heart. I wrap my body in white light to protect me when I'm afraid. I surround my children with white light when they go off to school. When I travel, I envelop the pilot and the plane in white light. I am very liberal in my use of the light of love. All of this is my conscious intent, to invoke divine love. Since I can't image love, I represent divine love with white light. I believe I have the choice to view any situation in my life either positively or negatively, and I choose to be affirmative about everything. I believe that everything can be redeemed in the light of love.

I have no contact with physicians. Even if I broke my arm, I would use a healer who sets breaks by manipulating contact points on the opposite limb.

I have such negative feelings about orthodox medicine that if I suspected I had cancer, I would go to great lengths to find an alternative way to deal with it. Although I admit there are certain circumstances where drugs and surgery have limited validity, I will say, however, that under no circumstances would I ever go to a hospital.

A healer I know is by training a chiropractor, but her treatments are based on diet and vitamins. She is also very psychic and she was very helpful to me. I went from her to my acupuncturist. I apply what I learn from healers to my entire family.

My biggest gripe is that doctors have no caring, no interest, no time. I'm treated like a thing and charged an exorbitant fee.

I recently saw a psychic about my physical health and received wonderful help from him. What he told me dovetails with my intuition and all the other health information sources I have. Everything must be checked out with my own perceptions. For example, the psychic reader recommended a particular dose of vitamin E which didn't seem right to me. After I tried it, I knew it was too much, and I halved the dosage. If I hadn't perceived that the larger amount would bother me, I'd have been uncomfortable for a few weeks. No health information can be followed blindly. My sensations are the real test. Whenever I have a psychic reading, it simply confirms what I already know at some other internal level. The psychic reading corroborates the truth, and somewhere in me, I know the truth.

One of my children has a recurring problem with eczema. When I took her to doctors all I ever got was a prescription for cortisone ointment. All that does is control the exzema, but the ointment doesn't deal with the cause. I dealt with this problem in two ways. I took my daughter to see the chiropractor I mentioned earlier and she suggested vitamin A. We increased the vitamin A intake and all the eczema cleared up. The causal agent was still unknown.

Next, we went to the acupuncturist and he diagnosed problems in one of my daughter's lungs. Apparently the lungs were not ade-

182

quately eliminating toxic material, and the skin had to take over. After a few acupuncture treatments the eczema vanished and has never returned. I don't believe that any doctor and his diagnostic tools would have found the cause of the eczema.

Ann is obviously a good illness manager, but, more important, she is able to use her own healing energy, or to act as an instrument for a higher power, to accomplish self-healing.

My next self-healing interview subject, Jan, is somewhat eclectic. She manages a wide range of health resources and is literally an architect of her own health as we will see. Jan's health resources range from a conventional health-maintenance organization (the Kaiser Foundation in California) to psychic readers. She speaks cautiously but well of her current relations with physicians. She says simply, "I know exactly what to expect of doctors, and they are always there when I need them."

Three of Jan's children were delivered at the Kaiser Foundation Hospital and she describes the events as "good experiences in spite of Kaiser's maternity methods." Her first child was delivered by a natural childbirth method in another setting. The three later births at Kaiser Hospital went so quickly that before the doctors were prepared the babies were there. Jan exudes delight when she recalls those moments. "The doctors had no time to give me drugs and the births were completely natural."

Fifteen years ago, Jan learned in natural childbirth training not to resist pain. It was a revelation to go with the pain and sense the difficulty subsiding, and she never forgot it.

Jan has seen the best and the worst of scientific medicine, and she has the stories to back up this claim. The beginning stages of tuberculosis were detected in her husband during a routine multiphasic physical examination. The subsequent treatment and hospitalization completely arrested the disease and blocked a death that would have been premature by two or three decades. Jan marvels at how well that medical episode was managed by conventional medicine.

On the other hand, Jan tells of her mother, who lived much of her life as a victim of her own physical condition. She bounced in and out of hospitals endlessly. When she was eight months pregnant with her fourth child she had gas pains which were diagnosed as appendicitis. An operation revealed a healthy appendix, but the side effects of the surgery, which occurred only a few weeks before term, were contributory to the baby's death shortly after birth. Based on Jan's current awareness of her own health, it is her contention that her mother had nutritional problems most of her life. Yet physicians never helped her with her diet.

Jan contends that all illness begins in minute signs which many people ignore, often out of a sense of false pride. If those small early signals are picked up, the aware person usually knows what is happening and any healer's diagnosis is only a verification.

Jan has spent a great deal of time developing and honing her self-awareness. The benefits of this steady effort are constantly evident. A few years ago she received a battery of tests for a suspected bladder infection. The results indicated that surgery was needed. She intuitively knew that "it didn't seem right." She returned to the doctor and asked that the complex, expensive tests be repeated. On the second run the results were negative—no infection was present. Checking back, the doctor was able to find a laboratory processing failure that caused the erroneous first results.

Jan puts it this way: "I go to doctors for diagnosis, but I would check many sources before I would ever have surgery. I'd see other doctors and I would get physical readings from psychics." But, she cautions, "Psychics have

184

off-days like anyone else, and they can get you into as much trouble as a regular doctor."

One of the most fascinating things Jan told me was her criteria for choosing a psychic to do a physical reading. In Chapter 2 I wrote of the difficulty of choosing a doctor. For most people simply locating a psychic reader would be a difficult task, but Jan has applied herself to that problem as to all other areas of her health. She sat relaxed in her chair and reviewed the qualities that are important to her.

I choose a psychic for a physical reading based on three things. First, I look at the general condition and apparent health of the psychic. If he is a chain smoker or his body is a disaster area, then I'm more cautious than I might otherwise be.

Next, I look at the extent to which they involve me in the reading. I want an interaction with them and I'm not asking them to prove themselves. I go knowing that these people are psychic, so I tell them everything I've learned, and let them take it from there. The reading itself must be a give-and-take between us.

The last quality of a psychic reader that is important to me is to determine how dogmatic they are. Do they take away my responsibility and not allow me to participate in my own healing? I want the psychic to act as a catalyst, to help me to see what I may not be sure of, and to give me verification of what I already know.

The first thing that Jan does whenever she suspects any physical problems is to check her nutritional state. She does this by having a biochemical analysis (see List 1 in Chapter 6). She merely touches her tongue to a piece of special paper, mails the paper to a laboratory, and in a short time she has an assessment of her body chemical balance. Jan believes that any organic disorder in the body is the result of chemical imbalances which precede the organic upset. The chemical imbalance may be the consequence of changing emotions, attitudes, or actual organic changes. "I'm paying attention to all these levels," she says. Working from the laboratory report, Jan will take the required "tissue salt" until her body chemistry is back in balance. We will return to this subject later in this chapter.

Jan recalled a recent experience with a chiropractor. For some time she had had a sense of uneasiness and slight discomfort. Something simply was not right. When Jan became surer that she wanted to get in touch with a healer, a chiropractor was recommended to her through friends.

When she visited the chiropractor, her intuition put a stamp of approval on his healing ability. She sensed, however, that his personal emotional state was uncertain, and that was an important realization. Jan has found that if a healer has personal problems, that negative energy will often spill over into his healing work. Awareness of this possibility allows Jan to block the "bad vibes." Jan's position is that, as a patient, she is responsible for everything, good or bad, that comes to her from a healer.

Jan conducted a careful transaction with the chiropractor. They made a specific agreement that he was to do certain work on her spine. She was concerned to find that he knew nothing about nutrition, and, before his work began, she took pains to see that they were both clear on exactly what was going to happen. At the time I talked with Jan she said that the chiropractor had been helping her.

Jan has cogent comments to make about her experience with large prepaid group practice plans such as Kaiser, where all of scientific medicine is brought together in a single location to create a kind of medical supermarket. In spite of the obvious merit of the arrangement, Jan contends that "you still have to do it yourself. Though referrals are given, you must know what you want and determine where to find it in that medical beehive."

Fringe medicine provides another medical bazaar and, as we have seen, there are few guidelines for finding your way around it. Jan knows that the responsibility for getting what she wants from this metaphysical market is hers. She increases her chances for success in self-healing by emphasizing three things. She has done a great deal of work on her emotional state so that she is in a fairly stable condition. She examines carefully her attitudes toward herself and other people. And last she pays a lot of attention to the food she eats and her nutritional state.

Jan deals with the buildup of tension in her life by spending time with herself. The sensitive awareness that Jan has of herself and the world around her has a complicated aspect. "One thing I'm trying to deal with now is that I am psychically open to a number of people in my life. To be open at that level means I'm open emotionally, too. I pick up my friends' stresses and experience whatever they are going through. If I know the negative feelings are coming from outside me, I can block them. Often, however, I can't separate the problems I'm picking up from my friends from my own difficulties. The more I know myself, the closer I am to making this distinction. In fact, I've learned that I protect myself in all ways by really knowing myself."

Jan says that, in a nutshell, self-healing is being able to tune in to yourself and knowing where to make lifestyle changes. The rationale for Jan's approach is the concept that each person has the option of creating a unique lifestyle based on his or her own perceptions. Formula living according to particular group styles is discarded for general flexibility.

One of the key external means that Jan uses to monitor her health is biochemical analysis, a method based on the existence of twelve tissue salts that were isolated by the physician W. H. Schuessler in 1873. He determined that these minerals are integral constituents of the body by identifying them in human blood as well as in the ashes of humans after death.

Schuessler determined by experimentation that if the body becomes deficient in these minerals, the deficiency causes an abnormal or diseased condition. He studied various symptoms and compared them to the minerals that were lacking in the persons he examined. It was his conclu-

187

sion that if the diseases he found were at all curable, and if the proper tissue salt were chosen and given in the correct amount, the deficiency which caused the abnormality was corrected and the body healed itself.

Mira Louise, the late Australian naturopath, found an interesting connection between radioactive fallout and tissue salts. Her work reads like science fiction. Radioactive fallout is carried from the stratosphere to earth by rain or snow, deposited in our soil, picked up by the plants we eat, and transferred to our bodies. When minor cases of radiation sickness have occureed, many types of symptoms are possible: low energy, falling hair, parched skin, eye trouble, skin rashes, headaches, and more. Mira Louise's theory was that the radiation sickness was actually due to bone and blood damage and the tissue salts are usually sufficient to restore health and vitality.

When I have asked physicians for their opinions of tissue salts, most have not heard of them. Two physicians who had heard of them thought of them only as "curiosities."

The number of persons I have met who call themselves self-healers and who are successful at it is small. Many people are in *transitional* stages in which combinations of self-awareness, the ability to relax, and deep intuition about coordinating other healer's work with their own personal efforts, are moving them toward some degree of self-healing.

There is a crucial element in developing the ability for self-healing. Basically, it involves being able to remain calm when the pressure is on. In modern psychological terms, this is called "being centered," which means having the ability to stay relaxed, to contain your energy and strength, and to retain all your problem-solving abilities when there is a crisis in your life.

I've heard physicians scoff at the notion of self-healing. One said to me, "Say what you will about fringe medicine and taking care of yourself, but just let a painful, frightening illness strike and then we'll see what you do. Ten to one you will run, not walk, to your family doctor."

Most of us have experienced what the doctor describes. We are so conditioned to present ourselves passively to a physician with our personal strengths—physical and psychological—depleted far beyond what is appropriate for the illness. Being "off center" in a doctor's office is the rule rather than the exception. The ability to remain centered during a crisis generally requires a great deal of personal development.

Linda is a woman who learned a great deal about healing long before she was emotionally capable of taking advantage of it.

She speaks with a highly controlled and carefully modulated voice. Each utterance seems like a mini-speech. Her awareness of herself as a teacher is expanding, and I felt it when I interviewed her.

She described her rather unhappy childhood. Raised by an older sister in a large family, Linda was able to get attention from her mother only by getting sick. This sickness pattern took years to detect and overcome. As a teenager, Linda was, in her words, "a rigid, tense, and highly controlled person."

When she was a young woman an unusual experience came her way. Through a friend she was invited to join a group of people who participated in faith-healing. Can you picture her? It's twenty years ago, she is an immature and anxious twenty-year-old, and she, along with the other members of her group, are acting as healing energy channels, in order to heal people.

She speaks of those days with warmth and enthusiasm. She was instructed to pray in the group and use the Christ-light to bathe the sick person in healing energy. She learned the dangers of becoming ill by involving herself with the person receiving the faith-healing.

Linda knows the power of group prayer, and she relates

189

stories of astonishing cures. But she became aware of a strange situation. There was a seemingly unbridgeable void between her life in the healing group and her everyday life. None of the healing skills and knowledge she acquired in the group seemed to go with her when she moved on with her own life. In recalling those days, she says, "I simply was not centered; I had so much work to do on myself."

Linda's holistic-healing path has been a long trial-and-error effort. She has been a vegetarian, has meditated, has developed her psychic ability, has belonged to therapy and encounter groups, has been rolfed, has been in bioenergetic therapy, and has gone through the Pecci-Hoffman process. This mixing of healing methods extended over several years. Most of her earlier life and part of this period as well have been characterized by generally poor physical condition and she has had several surgical operations.

There is no astounding punch-line to Linda's story. She is a holistically-minded person who is beginning to be able to self-heal after starting with the healing cart in front of the horse. There has been a steady improvement in the quality of her life. As her emotional problems, especially with her parents, have been resolved, the spiritual awareness of her early healing experiences has found a comfortable place in her life. She says, "As my self-awareness grew, I felt the direction of a higher being. I finally let my resistance go and said 'All right, I give up, Father. What is thy will?'"

Linda visualizes illness as a chain forged with three links. The first link is one's attitude or beliefs about some issue. The attitudes then affect emotional response during some event involving the issue; and the final link is the influence on the physical body.

I tested her theory by asking what she would do if she learned that heart trouble were imminent for her. "First," she said, "I would develop an attitude of very positive hope about the danger. I would convince myself that whatever was to happen was an experience to be accepted

190

and understood. I would gently inquire of myself how and why I arranged to have heart trouble. I would use every healer and health resource available that I sensed could help me."

There it is—attitude control. Self-healing is based on developing a positive attitude towards healing. Linda's use of physicians and drugs depends on her perception of what is happening. She suggests letting go of any belief system that claims, for instance, that all drugs are bad or that no doctor can do you any good.

Using some of the ideas presented in this chapter, let's look at the common cold. Hundreds of remarks like "We can put men on the moon but we can't cure the common cold" have been born because of the extraordinary resistance the cold offers to being cured.

The scientific description of a cold that a doctor uses goes something like this. Colds are caused by viruses which are tiny living things that reproduce only inside the cells of other organisms. The viruses seek out your respiratory system because the living is so good there—right levels of temperature, chemical content, moisture, and energy. These levels are controlled by messages from your mind. When conditions are right, the viruses move in and the body fights back. White blood cells and antibodies to kill the viruses are carried in by a surge of blood flow to the nose and throat, and mucus is produced to flush away the viruses. Fighting back, then, means a red, runny nose.

Other by-products of the battle are body chemicals that cause fever, tiredness, and multiple discomforts. All these symptoms are evidence that your body is getting on with the business of healing itself. If the battle is not successfully won very soon, the swollen, wet, mucus-covered tissue of your respiratory system becomes a marvelous home for the growth of bacteria, and more serious problems such as strep throat, bronchitis, and pneumonia may be next.

To recapitulate, both the presence of viruses and a proper living environment for them in your nose and throat are necessary for you to catch a cold. Though you can't see the viruses, runny noses and coughs signal their presence. To give them a hospitable place to survive, you must be out of harmony with yourself and nature. Things like tension, anxiety, unhappiness, poor nutrition, lack of rest and cleanliness, and tissues irritated by tobacco and other chemicals are possible contributors to creating the ground on which the viruses can flourish.

And now, the healing. As you sit there with your stuffy head, be aware that you have the power to heal yourself. You, your body and the viruses are a part of all other beings and elements that form the world. The cold is a message that there is some disharmony in your little corner of the world. Intuitively you will know how to make changes and strive for greater harmony.

The cold symptoms are a natural sedative, so slow down, don't resist the symptoms, just rest and relax. Surrender to the cold. As you give in to the cold, check your energy level. Is there something you should be doing, or someone for whom you want to be healthy, or is there a possibility that the cold prevents you from exploring?

These intuitive flashes back to your emotional state give clues to the sources of disharmony, and there will be as many different reasons as there are people.

As you rest and build your body's energy for combating the virus, find ways to relax so that in no way will your body slow blood flow or hinder the healing process. Relaxing will also ease those stiff muscles.

Be direct and intentional about it. Do a relaxation exercise. For example, mentally talk to the parts of your body. Ask your feet to relax and then continue, part by part, on up to your scalp. As you practice this exercise you can note the slowing and deepening of your breathing. If your physician were watching you, he could observe the tension going out of your muscles as you relaxed.

192

The learning that occurs in this type of self-healing will teach you to pay attention to activities and situations in your life that cause tension or put extra stress on your body and mind. By becoming aware of these conditions and reducing them you will diminish the frequency and severity of future occurrences.

I chose the cold as an obvious example of self-healing because there is no known cure in scientific medicine. Self-healing has the potential to fill the gap when other healers are not able to help.

Self-healing, which is evolving as patients explore themselves is still a slippery subject. Doctors seem confused by the concept of self-healing. Those I've talked with are instinctively attracted to the notion that patients can assume more responsibility for their health, but resist whenever specifics are mentioned. Do your own physical exam? Impossible. Have your baby at home with a midwife in attendance? Dangerous. Diagnose your own illness? Ridiculous. Treat yourself? Idiocy.

And one more question: Create your own doctor? Insane. Yes, that's what I said, "Create your own doctor." To be more accurate I should say imagine your own healer. Additional reading materials on this attractive idea are listed in the Chapter Notes. Just think about the advantages. Your imaginary doctor is available anytime you need him. He makes nothing but housecalls. Since he is a creation of your imagination, he is an instrument to ventilate and validate all those things you know about yourself, but never quite admit. Your doctor has the wisdom of a three-thousand-year-old healer. That's how long the body has had to learn to heal itself and your doctor possesses all of that knowledge. The idea is far from new. Many cultures, including the American Indians, have used "spirit guides" for healing. The contemporary Pecci-Hoffman therapy uses such a guide.

Instructions for creating your imaginary doctor are given in *The Well Body Book* by Samuels and Bennett.

There are four basic steps: relax, imagine a house, imagine a room in that house, meet and consult with your imaginary doctor in that room in the house.

If this sounds a bit strange to you, look at it this way: Have you ever had a trusted friend who was so close to you that he knew what you were thinking and feeling even when you found it difficult to articulate your thoughts and feelings? Such a friend responds to your deeper uncensored levels and may be called your alter ego. All of us have an alter ego or second self *within* us, a part of us that is not blocked by ego, pride, guilt and other surface feelings, but instead represents our inner core of being.

The imaginary doctor can be a helper or adviser to the real you when your actual friend isn't around. If you are being disabled by fear because of an illness, visit your imaginary doctor, who you can trust completely. Some people use their imaginary doctor for all kinds of problem solving—from finding a lost cat to arbitrating an argument with a friend. Whenever you feel anxious, confused, or doubtful and want to relax and work things out, the imaginary doctor can help you step back from those feelings and more clearly work on your problem. Yet the act of creating your imaginary doctor may require a kind of letting-go which eludes you. My only counsel is to "try easier." Your imaginary doctor may be an important part of your self-healing.

In many different ways it is clear that all healing is self-healing. Regardless of the treatment—a drug to change the metabolism, a psychologist to help a patient with deeply buried conflicts, an acupuncture treatment to remove blocks in the flow of vital energy—unless the patient *permits* the treatment to be beneficial, it is not likely that a permanent cure will result. Many healers have observed that often the patient, consciously or unconsciously, defeats the attempts of the healer. The patient's attitude of opposition to cure is generally deeply unconscious.

The practice of self-healing seems to require an optimistic view of life and the ability to draw on deeper and richer stores of energy from within oneself, rather than from without. Many external activities are helpful, such as care about food choice, exercises to keep the spine and muscles flexible, good breathing habits, and specific medical treatments. Ultimately, however, the essence of self-healing is the recognition that within each of us there lies an infinite source of power, peace, and psychic vitality upon which we can draw.

If we are working against the negative forces in our life represented by polluted air, high noise levels, toxic working conditions, and urban decay, the self-healing task is much more difficult. It is easier to stay healthy in some environments than in others.

In a highly antagonistic environment, energy flags, tempers get tender, and the "white light" darkens. Some element of self-will or self-repudiation, of subtle hatred or withdrawal, of self-interest or self-pity, has crept in. Depending on your own awareness, you may not detect the intruder until the psyche is subtly and insidiously poisoned. Finally, some physical symptom betrays you to yourself. That's the way a majority of illnesses occur. When and how you intervene is up to you.

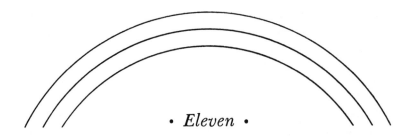

The Future

Americans in the 1970s are making the most fundamental life adjustments they have ever had to make. Forces have emerged which the prudent American takes to mean that life will never be the same again. From whatever angle you approach the issues, be it resources, inflation, population, or politics, the prognosis is the same. Solutions to our problems will require permanent alterations in the size and scope of our activities, possessions, and dreams.

At this point in the twentieth century, the feeling that best characterizes the lives of many people is tension. Consider the pressures of modern living. The inexorable rises in the cost of food, materials, services, and medical care. The problems of recession, unemployment, taxes, the energy crisis, and violence. The heightened sense of individual powerlessness that comes from fears of governmental abuses of power and burgeoning corporate power. The health hazards of additives in foods and chemicals in the environment. And the need to adapt to changing roles of men and women.

Indications of stress are everywhere. Books that offer clues to tapping the peace and tranquility buried within us become best sellers. Memberships in groups that offer

196

instruction in relaxation are booming. Sales of tranquilizers have never been higher. The demand for counseling has far outstripped the availability of mental health services.

It is from this milieu of the last two decades that the move toward holistic healing has appeared. Chance? I think not. A number of national energies have combined to produce it. The actors in this play are the patients, the medical professionals, and our institutions. Waiting anxiously in the wings, and hoping for at least a brief appearance, are the understudies, the metaphysicians who have no way to share the stage except by the power of their natural talents. How will the roles of the present major actors and the understudies evolve as the medical drama of the 1980s unfolds?

Ideally a healer's role is catalytic. Having particular knowledge and position, he or she should have and exercise the option of moving back and forth among other specialists and other situations, gathering facts and formulating new ideas and fresh policies. That statement should apply to any of our health professionals, but unfortunately rarely does. Their resistance to change is manifold.

The role of the healing professions should be to prevent violence and brutality to the human *body, mind, and spirit.* Violence and brutality are used in the most general sense and refer to actual life conditions and experiences that cause you to be unhealthy. Air pollution or a fight with a relative, for example. Or you may be brutalized by the policies of your local city council.

But the training of physicians is still based on a physician-patient relationship or confrontation where the patient is experiencing some already existing illness. It is this unrelenting focus on pathology that blocks a preventive approach to health. There is little effort to attack the roots of the violence and brutality. Most medical professional effort and research is solidly connected to dealing with a sick person. Yet a doctor could also fulfill the Hippocratic

Oath by deciding to study how many protuberances on an automobile's instrument panel can inflict a fatal would on a motorist's head.

Current academic conditions in medical schools are not encouraging. Holistic concepts receive little attention. The most innovative curriculum change now under debate is a reversal of the specialist-versus-generalist pendulum swing. Remember the family doctor who tried to do everything for you? Those generalists faded away and were replaced by platoons of pathological specialists. Medical leadership eventually realized specialization had gone too far and called for a return of the generalist. After great effort the general practitioner is coming back, but wearing the professionally acceptable cloak of yet another specialty—"family practice."

The existent value structures of the medical profession strongly influence the development of doctors who are not interested in the problems of hunger and malnutrition or the violent technology implicit in unsafe consumer products. Silent violence like air and water pollution gets little attention. It is a sad testimonial to present-day professional values that the more untreatable and rare is the disease specialty, the higher the status of the corresponding medical discipline.

Most healers, working by whatever guidance or influence, choose to treat only the last events (symptoms) in a long chain of causality. The most abhorred offender should be the healer whose healing efforts suppress symptoms that themselves are part of natural healing processes.

Our national resources are allocated to a sociology of diseases which includes a priority list. Polio once received and now sickle cell anemia is receiving a great deal of attention while diseases that ravage far greater numbers of people, such as arthritis, are ignored.

It is clear that the medical profession needs a full-time, high-status role for physicians who are not working in hospitals or in clinics, and who do not deal with patients, but who deal with managing such things as the allocation of resources in a society, and the legal system under which technology is developed.

Salaried industrial physicians are a classic case in point. As poor cousins of the medical profession, they are constantly told that they cannot publish their case data. Consumer advocate Ralph Nader has written of a physician at a beryllium plant in Cleveland who had a number of case studies on beryllium poisoning, but was blocked from publishing it. There are unacceptable, out-of-vogue, and censored areas of study, research, and publication in every professional society, medical societies included. It is inappropriate here to examine the details of this massive subject except to point out the grandfather of them all: You have only to look at the allocations in the Federal budget to see what gets attention in our society. The professional who deviates, from publication guidelines, say, loses privileges and may become a pariah. Many of the standards of the medical profession have the effect of defeating the right of dissent.

We need health professionals who can overcome stifling restrictions and are free to advocate, are free to investigate, free to testify, free to propose dramatic solutions that may have economic impact, and free to cut vested interests away from the development of medical technology.

Of course, the majority of my comments are directed to the most organized health professional of all, the physician. Unfortunately, other healers, such as osteopaths and the chiropractors, who have achieved a degree of social and professional acceptance, are emulating many of the negative professional activities of the doctors; for example, the near impossibility of getting one health professional to evaluate another one. Another example is the area of occupational health and safety. Cases like the beryllium poisoning just mentioned constitute a social malaise that is at least three times as serious as street crime in this country in terms of required facilities, trauma, and the incidence of related disease. Physicians are only peripherially involved in this area, and national priorities look the other way.

Patients of today are concerned about preventive medicine. We all have wearied of a professional health industry that is basically an illness system. We are asking for care before we get sick, not after. This is so important that we must take the point to the healers themselves.

Talking to physicians about prevention can turn up some surprises. One point of view was stated by H. E. Emerson in a recent issue of the *Journal of the Canadian Medical Association.*

Suppose we take the indices of mortality in our society: arteriosclerotic disease and cancer head the list. We know that arteriosclerosis is linked with high protein, high fat diet, with cigarette smoking, with overweight and under-exercise, and probably with the sort of stress engendered on the one hand by being a Minister of Health, or on the other hand by being one of the objects of his execration. What can we, the physicians, do about these things? We have given our advice to our patients, who are our masters, and to our political masters, who are also sometimes our patients. We cannot force them to cut their protein, fat and carbohydrate intake to optimal levels, to quit their cigarettes, to walk instead of ride, or to cease from making or listening to the sort of statements calculated to cause stress; to live, in summary, godly, righteous and sober lives. . . . We have told them (the politicians) and our patients what they should do to be healthy. How can we—or should we—make them do it? We know that in Vienna and Amsterdam from 1940 to 1945 the death rate from arteriosclerotic disease fell precipitously; does our community want, in return for this sort of amelioration, to adopt that sort of diet? And is it our job to enforce it?

Later in the same article, Dr. Emerson wrote:

On the one hand we have knowledge of preventive medicine which is not applied because of governmental inertia, or disinterest, or bureaucratic boondoggles, and on the other hand we have know-

200

ledge which is not applied because of personal preference, social pressure, or what you will. We have *in toto* too little knowledge about prevention, about the causes of morbidity as opposed to mortality, and frequently within medicine we have a hidebound approach and a dedication, not so much to tradition, as to the customary narrow paths to which our tunnel vision blinkers us.

Emerson says the problem with preventive medicine is the patients, the doctors, the politicians, and the culture. Discouraging.

Chogla is also a healer and he has a solution to Dr. Emerson's quandary on the other side of the healing spectrum. He belongs to the Teton Dakota Tribe on the Oglala Reservation in South Dakota. Chogla is a shaman and he heals a wide variety of major and minor mental and physical illnesses. He has always wanted to have a cooperative practice with the physicians of the U.S. Public Health Service, but it has never happened. Arrangements can be made with Chogla to have a healing ceremony to deal with future illnesses—in other words, preventive medicine. Such a healing is called a "catch the stone" ceremony. All who have contact with the ceremony are said to receive its benefits.

In the evening the healer, the patient, and any guests assemble in the healer's house and the doors and windows are covered with blankets. In the kerosene lamplight the shaman places paper on the floor and forms on it a small altar of earth, which he smooths flat and inscribes with his forefinger in a pattern of lines and dots. Offerings include colored cloth, a ball of rawhide cord, a bowl of water, braided sweetgrass, and a medicine pipe. The symbols on the altar are changed and sprinkled with tobacco while the shaman prays. Eagle feathers and two rawhide rattles are then placed upon the altar.

Next, the shaman lights the sweetgrass and waves the smoke about the room as the lamp is turned out. A long period of rattling sounds, prayers, songs, and drumming follows. Spirit powers are invoked and flashes of light (from a flint-steel wheel?) are seen. Seemingly endless prayers ensue, with the healer's voice rising and falling, interspersed with howling, prolonged songs, flashing sparks, hooting sounds, grunts, cries, and continued rattling.

Suddenly all of this stops, and a shrill voice, apparently coming from the shaman, invokes references to all dead relatives of the patient. The lamp is lighted and the healer points dramatically to the altar where a black "spirit stone" has appeared. The stone, wrapped in buckskin and tied to a necklace-length cord, is presented to the patient to protect her always against illness and danger. She is told that if disease or injury threatens, she will be awakened in the night by spirits and given verbal warnings.

The ceremony ends with a meal of dogmeat, fried bread, berry pudding, and coffee.

Such protective amulets are nothing new, but viewed in the context of preventive medicine, especially if they are meant to guard body, mind, and spirit, they are more impressive.

In the comments quoted above, Dr. Emerson assumed that preventive efforts should be aimed at protecting only the body. He declared that the patient would not do what he should do. The shaman, on the other hand, implied by his every action that he would do it all for the patient. Neither attitude will produce what I continue to dream of: a relationship between patient and healer in which good health is constantly maintained and illness is always dealt with at very early stages. That will require the development of new roles for our healers and new perceptions of old roles.

How do we develop new roles for our health professionals? The problems of professional constraints, the lack of cooperation and support among healers, and false status symbols are woven into the fabric of our society and role

202

changes are difficult and threatening to those who try them. If any healer seriously explores the chain of causality that preceded the symptoms of the typical patient, it is likely he will be trespassing on at least one other professional's ground. Mind, body, and spirit are kept in separate compartments in the professions and academic disciplines and in the role definitions of our culture. There are dangers associated with violating that separateness. Somehow healers, health professionals, and institutions must recognize that compartmentalized professional relevance has little meaning when you are dealing with human health problems.

There are a few interdisciplinary settings where physicians, lawyers, scientists, and others are working in public interest areas such as health and contributing from both their specialized roles and their citizen roles. The major difficulty is money. Even if problems of role definition and interlocking roles are overcome, there still is no source of generalized financial support for interdisciplinary effort in our economic system. The traditional distinctions between mind, body, and spirit are still part of the funding criteria of institutions.

Most health professionals adjust to the role defined for them, and patients who are aware of this limitation must find ways to circumvent it. We need more individuals and training environments that place emphasis on a human's overall potential and the options that are available.

In the absence of change, must the patient take on the role of victim? In the preceding pages we have heard from many people who will not listen passively and take what is given, but want a more active role.

But in a broader context the patient is a *consumer* of health services, with problems not unlike those of any other consumer. Ralph Nader wrote the following in a recent article:

The most important new development in medicine, quite apart from the National Health Insurance, quite apart from the basic issues

203

of cost control and quality control and capacity of delivery is, I think, the role of the consumer in the restructuring of medical care. This is going to take a lot of ego friction to overcome. It is going to have to develop a great deal of humility within the professions, and within other professions as well. It is going to, in effect, challenge the canons of ethics, not just in terms of verbal challenges, appeals to the oath or to the legal canon of ethics or the engineering canon of ethics, but to bring the canons into straight collision with power. That is the only way that they are going to be utilized instead of eulogized.

The people whose holistic healing experiences have appeared in this book have attempted to manage their own health. They are the pioneers in a new social-medical consciousness and can serve as models to others. Their health successes have been due largely to the sharpness of their own intuition and awareness. Their stories make useful information available to others and show that hard positions regarding healing can be softened, and that people's healing realities can be changed. The people described in this book have placed a high priority on internal events and inner development. Each person has progressed along lines that are consistent with his or her motivation and interest. As future generations of such questing patients experience even rudimentary forms of holistic medicine, more will be learned. These patients, by their own choice, are research subjects gathering information for themselves and others. Ultimately, this may be the greatest contribution an individual can make.

I see no clear separation between so-called growth activities and whole-body healing experiences and I made no such distinction. As we have seen, the spectrum of choice available for individual activity ranges from various scientific medical practices to analytical psychology, from the humanistic and transpersonal disciplines to the most esoteric concepts of mysticism. In spite of the overpowering breadth of these options, they all have closely related purposes. They achieve those purposes by different means. Each in its own way and within its own limits reveals to you the nature of your body and your psyche; and many hint at your relation to the universe.

Short-run attempts at experiencing holistic healing may produce very different results depending on the path you take. The book, teacher, therapist, healer, group leader, hypnotist, or guru will help you move towards the integration of a healthy body, mind, and spirit by facilitating the healing of the parts that they can contact. It will be up to you to determine which paths you choose to follow and where you will be when you get to a healthy state as defined by you. No one can tell you. Many people limit their health expectations to the condition of their body. It never occurs to them to attempt to evolve in mind or spirit.

Much has been written about the different levels of human consciousness, but there is no general agreement on the definition of any state of consciousness. A person's state of consciousness seems to set the level of healing expectation. There is something in certain people which urges them to seek better states of health. No one has identified this factor, but in a simplistic empirical fashion I can identify three evolutionary steps which lie beyond a so-called normal level.

The first stage of evolution is seen in persons who recognize the power of their subconscious and want to control it primarily so they can perform better in the material world. They realize that control over their health state, especially their emotions and other subconscious functions, will improve their interpersonal experiences, work performance, and the like. They will do those things that relieve anxieties and eliminate annoying hang-ups. Often they learn self-hypnosis and other forms of mental control in order to improve their concentration and regulate their emotions.

Other people, higher on my evolutionary scale, accept the material world but look upon it in a different way. They see it as a place for experience and enjoyment, and they recognize the spiritual and mystical nature of the universe. Every moment of living is savored as a divine gift.

Still others, at the highest level of all, view the world as a dream-like illusion from which they wish to awaken. Divine consciousness is their goal.

You will note that the three categories imply a hierarchy of consciousness in which spiritual health is regarded as the most desirable state. This point is verified by almost all of the people I interviewed for this book. Where are you on this health ladder? There can be no single answer to the question that will fit everyone. It is likely that each reader will have different motivation and capacity and will aspire to different goals. The fact that you are reading this book suggests that you are responding to some internal or external guidance and that personal health evolution is desirable to you.

For most people a move toward whole-body healing begins with the cleaning out of personal garbage. The self-help health books will make a myriad of suggestions, a therapist or group leader will make more, and a spiritual teacher may require the greatest sacrifices of all. Money, time, energy, repetitious practice, and endless patience for being in the student role may be required to improve your holistic health state. Being open to new information and experience is a key attribute.

C. W. Henderson suggests self-hypnosis as a good starting point. He writes:

> If you want a dramatic exposure to your subconscious, self-hypnosis is a good starter. It's a striking demonstration of the power of your hidden psyche. It can enhance your life in the workaday world too, by improving your memory, your concentration or your self-discipline. And it can help in spiritual pursuits by allowing you to shift more easily from "normal" to altered states of consciousness, something that usually comes through conditioning built up over years of practice.

I suggest some kind of group experience as an alternate way to begin holistic healing. The details of the setting are not important as long as the basic ingredients of people being open, honest, and offering feedback are present. Many people have told me that when they learned how the world saw them that generated the motivation for development. That's an external trigger. For many others, the beginning experience is internal. A failure. Some kind of personal, social, or professional debacle starts the personal exploration.

Whatever the catalyst, and whatever their path to holistic healing, most people shop around at first. There are almost infinite combinations of techniques and philosophies to suit any personality. In the absence of a strong intuitive direction, it is wise to learn as much as you can about any individual healing alternative. Give your perceptions something to work on.

The sense of who you are as a person is with you always. The removal of the layers over you can be a life-long experience. The most important thing individuals can do about holistic healing is to start experimenting when the urge is there.

What sort of *institution* could facilitate the evolution of the practice of holistic medicine? Only a few experiments exist at the time of this writing. For the foreseeable future most individuals must manage their own synthesis of healers.

The greatest block to a holistic approach for large numbers of our population is the breach between traditional physicians and the rest of the healers. Holistic-healing clinics, in which all healers coordinate and cooperate to provide whole-body healing to individuals, exist only in our fantasies. The October 11, 1975, issue of the Los Angeles *Times* included an article that described plans for such a coalition, but it was to occur in a foreign setting and only for reasons that are extremely practical. The setting was to be rural Africa; the reasons, the shortage of scientific healers and the high cost of the existing health services. That plan is now under development by the World Health Organization of the United Nations with the intent of giving village healers some training in Western medicine. In effect, the program is turning local medicine men into paramedics and the practicing midwives into trained nurse-midwives. They are being taught to recognize and refer all serious cases to physicians. It is not the holistic healing collaboration I dream of, but if the program is successful, it may be a small move in the right direction.

Dr. Armin Geller, A French physician working in the Congo, says, "Most Africans now get whatever medical care they receive from the native practitioners. In a typical village there are even specialists: the herbalist, the bonesetter, the midwife, the psychiatrist. It is possible to utilize there people and make their work more relevant to modern medicine. Some countries in Africa average $1.00 per person per year for health care, and the minimum shots to prevent the main diseases cost $1.10 per person."

So far, most of the available medical funds have been spent either in showcase hospitals in big cities or in community hospitals and clinics in the smaller cities and larger towns. But the majority of Africans still *live* in villages. Nevertheless, though the plan is based solely on economic conditions, I suspect that the doctors and the village healers will ultimately learn a great deal from each other.

Dr. Harold Wise has proposed a holistic-healing clinic for families, which he calls "The Family Center." The following is from his statement of intention:

The Family Center will be dedicated to working on the whole health of a community of families, bringing medical skill to illness, psychological skill to distress, and human concern to the process of people becoming more fully functioning. The staff will be committed to helping the Center's clients unfold their own strengths to prevent, resist, and recover from disease. We will focus on preparing

208

people to manage effectively the major life transitions: birth, adolescence, marriage, mid-life change, retirement, and old age and dying—the critical events that have such impact on family life. We will also examine the working through of such unexpected life changes as illness, sudden moves, unemployment, and divorce. We will explore ways in which family members can be more supportive to each other as each individuates and develops.

Dr. Wise sees this as a step forward for holistic medicine in that the healing of the individual is viewed in the context of his immediate community, whether it is a family or a network of friends. Further, each "family" will be dealt with in *anticipation* of a series of identifiable life crises. And, most impressive of all, The Family Center intends to develop strategies to help the family prepare for times of multiple individual crises.

Dr. Wise gives as an example of multiple individual crises "a father in his forties, in a stressful job, who bears the accumulated effects of indoor work; his adolescent son coping with a changing body, explosive sensuality, and peer group pressure; a mother also in her forties, who has had the complex roles of wife and mother and is adjusting to the departure of the children and her need to establish a new form of intimacy with her husband; and a grandmother in her seventies, recently widowed, whose physical energies must be conserved in ordinary activities and who must face the crisis of dying."

The proposed Family Center is an extremely exciting and ambitious enterprise. It recognizes health as a complex matter. The medical structure will be based on a primary-care physician and nurse-practitioner being assigned to each family, backed up by a group of nutritionists, acupuncturists, family therapists, meditation teachers, and potentially a wide range of healers. The team of healers will work in collaboration with each family, for, as Dr. Wise says, "We feel the client is responsible for his organism, and our work is to help him find the resources for self-healing and unfoldment from within."

209

The Family Center will also have a research orientation. Experiments will attempt to determine those conditions most conducive to caring, healing, and individual development. The environment of the center is intended to be warm, personal, and non-clinical even though all appropriate medical and technical equipment will be available. The facilities are described this way: "Mineral baths, massage rooms, equipment for bio-feedback training, meditation space and room for jogging, aerobic dancing, and yoga will be available to the client families as part of their program for preventing disease and for expanding their sense of self."

The Family Center is planning a substantial educational program. Instruction in nutrition, breathing, body relaxation, bio-feedback, and other forms of self-development are mentioned in the proposal. Preventive healing will be emphasized by exploring hopes, expectations, needs, and plans in advance of life crises. The objective is to convert a family crisis into a growth experience.

The therapies to be provided by the center are also described in the proposal. "One major job of the permanent staff will be to continue to look at unorthodox systems, evaluate their effectiveness, and integrate those that seem valuable into the Center's treatment and development program. Some therapies we will consider initially are oriental medicine (acupuncture, herbalism, physical therapy), awareness therapies (Gestalt, psychosynthesis, body therapies, bio-feedback, Alexander method, bioenergetics, structural integration), therapeutic massage, and meditation."

I like the concept of the Family Center. It takes the idea of the individual holistic healer and moves it several steps ahead toward preventive holistic healing of the family. The Center is only a dream now, however. Whether it can happen in our culture at this time seems doubtful. It is a long step from the current discussions of national health insurance and health maintenance organizations to a holistic healing center. Individual patients are indeed working out their versions of holistic healing, but I predict that institutionalization like the Family Center will be a long time in coming.

A potential criticism of holistic healing as described in this book is that the participating individuals become intensely preoccupied with themselves. An essential inward-turning is required, to be sure. Carried to an extreme, the focus on the "I" could block the development of society. At shorter range, families, groups, and institutions are all weakened by the strong, individualistic, apparently selfish, inward-looking person.

Dr. Leonard Duhl of the University of California suggests that the family in any form: nuclear, extended, or even tribal, is essential for survival and for ultimate development of our society, which raises the question: can a holistically healthy person participate in any form of a family? Dr. Duhl writes of "holistic development" where healing is but one dimension.

Development to an optimal state, even for an individual, requires a relationship over time. A "family" is such a relationship, for it permits different people to be held together by a glue which assists growth as well as further individuality. It offers a chance for balance, for experiencing males and females, different generations and different views. A family can be destructive, oppressive, or even exploitive. However dangerous, a family still presents opportunities for development which an individual cannot make or have alone.

Therein, I believe, lies the next step. The holistically healthy person will not be a stoic alone on a mountain top, but will be actively involved, not only in a family, but in all cultural groups of our society. Holistic development involves all of the most fundamental aspects of body, mind, and spirit. Dr. Duhl continues:

I suggested the word "development" was critical. Within each of these areas, whether physical or psychological or spiritual, seem to be normal developmental processes. Anna Freud suggested some years ago that when various processes are out of synchronicity, issues such as illness evolve. When, in my words, mediation occurs between various aspects of development and they become synchronous, a more healthy activity occurs.

Duhl speculates that the *critical* factor is the *balanced* development of physical, psychological, emotional, and spiritual resources. He recognizes that in spite of the fact that many of the individuals who simulate holistic healing have their successes, little is known about how to put together the various pieces to fulfill the unique needs of any individual, family, or group. This agrees with our earlier observation that people proceed primarily on their own intuition. How do we deal with the inner and outer self? How do we reconcile individualism and aloneness versus conformity and belonging?

Duhl, like Wise, sees the transition or response periods following crisis as critical and proposes the establishment of Re-Creation Centers, where people in transition can come for assistance.

The Re-Creation Center (RC) will offer a place to retreat from the usual pressures of the world, and a setting to draw upon healing resources. Like Dr. Wise's Center, the RC would assist people in transition: divorce, change of job, death in the family, conflict with a friend, and so on. The RC would offer a setting for asking questions and elucidating issues as opposed to trying to determine specific solutions.

Dr. Duhl describes the RC this way:

A true Re-Creation Center is not eclectic nor laissez faire. It combines what is known with an awareness of where people are in their development, and starting there, facilitates a set of processes, using all modalities from the cognitive and rational, to the muscles, to the unconscious and the spiritual. What is striking is that each of us has different methods and modes by which to achieve states of change. I find it extremely difficult to reach those kinds of states in an individual meditative moment without interaction with signifi-

212

cant others. Some of these interactions are intellectual; but more often the issues involved in the process of creation for me are comradeship as in the national social programs, the civil rights movement, or Peace Corps where eating, sleeping, singing, and sharing were as important as doing, or the rational processes.

Any holistic set of development methods in an RC would recognize that people start from different backgrounds, have different patterns of response, and relate to different techniques in different order.

People who come to the RC would negotiate their own contracts of activities with the staff. It might include special nutrition, exercise, manual labor, massage, medical treatment, mental therapy, health education, group encounters, dance, music, art, and so on. A way to integrate a person's activities in the RC would be found in consultation with the staff. The RC sounds like a magical place, though its form, location, and staffing would be extremely difficult to accomplish today, and the exact nature of the groups and institutional activities is only the subject of fantasy today. Yet surely it is the future of holistic medicine. As Dr. Duhl writes, "Life is then a wholeness, a holiness, and a healthiness."

The Wholistic Health Center in Hinsdale, Illinois, is a church-based family practice medical care facility that combines physicians, pastoral counselors, and nurses to focus on all aspects of an individual's health. Their philosophical approach—holistic medicine—uses traditional healing professionals and compassionate volunteers to help the patients with all that is plaguing their lives at a given moment.

Dr. John Travis at the Wellness Resource Center in Mill Valley, California, looks at wellness, not illness, holistically. He wants to see you when you are feeling good, then he counsels you on nutrition, physical awareness, stress reduction, and self-responsibility so you can stay that way.

Let us go back now and discuss more fully the future of

213

holistic medicine at the state just beyond where most people who have appeared in this book seem to be. We have looked closely at people who have rebelled against the philosophical and clinical orientation that essentially dismisses all emotional and spiritual factors in disorders and considers both disease and health maintenance to be based upon purely physical considerations.

On the other side of the coin, however, criticism from our health professionals is leveled at the holistic healers. They are charged with promotion of the idea that all pathology is due to a "lack of self-awareness" on the part of the afflicted individual. Obviously, neither extreme is likely to be correct. The fact that such criticism is coming from the established health profession, however, indicates the need for a serious look at previously unconsidered research that has been swept aside because of role distinctions, over-specialization, and misplaced priorities. And much new research is needed. After all, what we all want as patients is a holistic medicine which is capable of dealing with the whole person and accounting for the inextricable interaction between that person and his environment. Although there is an extensive literature substantiating the idea of a disorder-prone personality, ways of averting these influences remain essentially unexplored. Examples are the Type A person who is predisposed toward heart trouble, and the carcinogenic person who is likely to develop cancer when subjected to extreme stress. People are waiting for holistic preventive health care, and the beginnings of pressure to acquire the appropriate knowledge and conditions are being felt. This book is meant to be part of that pressure. A ground swell of change in people's healing belief systems is building. The medical establishment is being asked to pay attention and to get involved in building a new health reality. Change in *national* healing beliefs is essential if there is to be any alteration in the allocation of national health resources,

214

because a natural characteristic of any system of belief is self-perpetuation: what is expected is observed and what is observed confirms the expectations.

I have no doubt that there are many instances in which traditional healing practices are a necessity, but it is also clear that stress disorders have long since replaced infectious diseases as our major health problem. Western medicine needs to explore the capacities of the mind to exert influences on a person's reaction to all kinds of illness.

The word consciousness has appeared frequently in these pages. Consciousness, awareness of something within oneself, is a primary force of life. Evidence of this is seen in the potential of visualization, hypnosis, dreams, and meditation in healing. Nevertheless, this concept of consciousness represents a belief change for many people.

Bear in mind that the changing of belief systems and the creation of even an individual new health reality are massive tasks requiring nearly a total personal energy investment for most people—at least at the start. I have seen people drop out, divorce, abandon responsibilities, and ignore their environment while pursuing holistic health. But if these phases are passed through, rebirth and new forms of healthy life are on the other side.

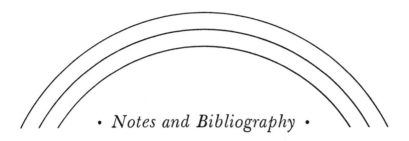

· *Notes and Bibliography* ·

Chapter 1: A RETURN TO HIPPOCRATES

Rene Dubos and Brian Inglis are the major influences on this chapter. Dr. Dubos, Professor Emeritus of Rockefeller University, is a microbiologist and experimental pathologist who first demonstrated the feasibility of obtaining germ-fighting drugs from microbes over forty years ago. He has long been intensely concerned with the effects that environmental forces—physicochemical, biological, and social—exert on human life. His *Mirage of Health* (New York: Harper & Row, 1971) is essential for the serious reader. Other writings by Dubos include *Man Adapting* (New Haven: Yale University Press, 1965) and *So Human an Animal* (New York: Charles Scribners' Sons, 1968).

Fringe Medicine by Brian Inglis (London: Faber and Faber, 1964) is an excellent example of a book on this medical topic by a European writer. European health professionals and patients are generally far more involved in and accepting of "fringe medicine" than Americans.

Perhaps the best known and most prolific author of historical writings on medicine was Henry E. Sigerist. Embedded in his many volumes, for example, *Civilization and Disease* (Chicago: University of Chicago Press, 1962), the persistent reader will find much valuable information about the evolution of scientific medicine.

Chapter 2: THE HEALER'S RITUAL

My statement on page 15 that "three-quarters of all ailments go away by themselves under fair conditions" has provoked considerable comment among advance readers of my text, so additional comment and explanation may be in order. Health planners differentiate between the *need* for medical services and the *demand* for them. In the past several decades the demand for medical services in most developed countries has grown to the extent that medical service facilities are frequently flooded. Most people used to stay home with a cold—now they see a doctor. Minor problems like short-term upper respiratory infections were once tolerated, now patients want symptom relief. Because of this, and because of a better understanding today of psychosomatic complaints, most medical authorities estimate the number of patients who will not get well by themselves to be less than a quarter of those who see doctors. Henry Bieler, M.D., in his book *Food Is Your Best Medicine* (New York: Random House, 1965), puts the figure at 20 per cent. It is obviously a difficult value to measure. The phenomenon of self-recovery is described well in *Magical Medicine: A Nigerian Case Study* by Una Maclean (New York: Penguin Books, 1974).

Again, since many readers will have taken antibiotics for viral infections, my statement on page 21 about antibiotics having no value in curing viruses may require explanation. It is true that to date no research has demonstrated that any antibiotic is successful in combating any virus. Other drugs are effective, but not antibiotics. The confusion arises because physicians frequently prescribe an antibiotic in case bacterial complications develop. Bacterial pneumonia is an example.

The comment by Lester Breslow on page 25 is from *Time,* December 23, 1974.

Understanding an African's experience of illness is important in softening our certainty regarding Western medicine. The British have had many health professionals involved in Africa for a very long time. The following list of works that may be of interest in connection with this chapter therefore contains a number of British titles.

Adler, H. M., and Hammett, V. O., "The Doctor-Patient Relationship Revisited," *Annals of Internal Medicine,* Vol. 78, 1973, pp. 595–598.

Alpert, J. J., "Slave Patients and Free Physicians," *New England Journal of Medicine,* Vol. 284, No. 12, March 25, 1971, pp. 667–668.

Gelfand, M., *Medicine and Custom in Africa* (London: E. & S. Livingstone, Ltd., 1964).

Haggard, H. W., *Devils, Drugs, and Doctors* (New York: Harper & Brothers, 1929).

Harley, G. W., *Native African Medicine* (London: Frank Cass & Co., Ltd., 1970).

King, S. H., *Perceptions of Illness and Medical Practice* (New York: Russell Sage Foundation, 1962).

Read, Margaret, *Culture, Health, and Disease* (London: Tavistock Publications, Ltd., 1966).

Todd, J. W., "The Errors of Medicine," The Lancet, 1:895, March 28, 1970.

Chapter 3: METAPHYSICAL HEALING

Sometimes it seems as though our culture is frozen in time and space. As a pragmatic nation we often ignore the learning of earlier times and information from other cultures. I have found that wide reading in anthropology and the history of medicine has given me a better perspective on contemporary health problems.

Several of the anthropological examples given in this chapter are based on research by Joan Halifax.

Many of the topics in the chapter were suggested by the following works:

Aleksandrowicz, Malca, "The Art of a Native Therapist," *Menninger Clinic Bulletin,* Vol. 36, 1972.

Bergman, R., "A School for Medicinemen," paper presented at the Annual Meeting of the American Psychiatric Association, Dallas, Texas, May 1972.

Bowers, J. K., "Hypnotic Aspects of Haitian Voodoo," *Journal of Clinical and Experimental Hypnosis,* 9:269, 1961.

Cannon, W. B., "Voodoo Death," *American Anthropology,* 44:169, 1942.

Clark, Margaret, *Health in the Mexican-American Culture,* 2nd Ed. (Berkeley: University of California Press, 1970).

Devereux, G., "Normal and Abnormal: The Key Problem of Psychiatric Anthropology," in Casagrande and Gladwin (Eds.), *Some Uses of Anthropology* (Anthropological Society of Washington).

Eliade, M., *Shamanism: Archaic Techniques of Ecstasy* (New York: Pantheon Books, Bollingen Series LXXVI, 1964).

Galdston, Iago (Ed.), *Man's Image in Medicine and Anthropology* (New York: International Universities Press, 1963).

Halifax-Grof, J., "Interaction Between Indigenous Healing and Contemporary Medicine," paper presented at the Annual Conference of the American Academy of Psychotherapists, New York, October 1972.

Harwood, A., "The Hot-Cold Theory of Disease," *JAMA,* 216:1153, 1971.

Jayne, W. A., *The Healing Gods of Ancient Civilizations* (New York: AMS Press, Inc., 1976; reprint of 1925 ed.).

Kiev, Ari, "The Psychotherapeutic Aspects of Primitive Medicine," *Human Organization,* 21, 1962.

Lester, D., "Voodoo Death: Some New Thoughts on an Old Phenomenon," *American Anthropology,* 74:386, 1972.

Middleton, John (Ed.), *Magic, Witchcraft, and Curing* (Austin: University of Texas Press, 1976).

Rogler, L. H., and Hollingshead, A. B., "The Puerto Rican Spiritualist as a Psychiatrist," *American Journal of Sociology,* Vol. 67, 1961.

Thorwald, J., *Science and Secrets of Early Medicine: Egypt, Babylonia, India, China, Mexico, Peru* (New York: Harcourt Brace Jovanovich, 1963).

Chapter 4: SCIENTIFIC MEDICINE

The intent of most current writings on health issues is to dispel three myths about health care. These myths are:

1. If we know the agent of a disease, then we know what causes the disease and how to prevent it.

2. If a population lives in undesirable circumstances, then their first health need is medical care.

3. Modern health care is the top priority need for all societies and has been responsible for the significant decrease in mortality rates and the population explosion.

All of these myths assume that any health care will be based on scientific medicine. The need to deal with these myths, difficulties in the delivery of health services, and concern about understanding the relationship between health and medicine have led to a flood of books in recent years, many of them polemical in tone and not very helpful. The most useful material for this chapter came from sources such as those listed below and from medical journals such as *New England Journal of Medicine.*

Lave, Judith, and Lave, Lester, "Medical Care and Its Delivery: An Economic Appraisal," *Law and Contemporary Problems,* 1970, pp. 252–266.

Luy, Mary Lynn, "How Will Medical Practice Change in the Next Decade?," *Modern Medicine,* Vol. 44, No. 1, January 1976, pp. 56–60, 63–66.

Perkins, David, and Thompson, John, "Assessment of Physicians' Attitudes Toward Community Health," *Community Mental Health Journal,* Vol. 10, No. 3, 1974, pp. 282–291.

Strauss, Anslem L. (Ed.), *Where Medicine Fails,* 2nd Ed. (New Brunswick, N.J.: Transaction Books, 1973).

Tancredi, L. R., and Barsky, A. J., "Technology and Health Care Decision Making," *Medical Care,* Vol. 12, No. 10, October 1974, pp. 845–859.

Chapter 5: THE MIND-BODY CONNECTION

The *mind-body* interface is the most studied of all possible combinations of two taken from *mind-body-emotions-spirit,* which is the connection we really want to know about, yet even of *mind-body* we know little. The following references offer examples of all we do know at this time:

Dunbar, Flander, *Mind and Body: Psychosomatic Medicine* (New York: Random House, 1947).

Grinker, R. R., *Psychosomatic Research* (New York: W. W. Norton, 1953).

Hamilton, Max, *Psychosomatics* (New York: John Wiley, 1955).

Hammond, S., *We Are All Healers* (New York: Harper & Row, 1973; Ballantine, 1974).

Jonas, Gerald, *Visceral Learning* (New York: Viking Press, 1973; Pocket Books, 1974).

Karagulla, Shafica, *Breakthrough to Creativity* (Los Angeles: De Vorss & Co., 1967).

Lewis, H. R., and Lewis, M. E. *Psychosomatics* (New York: Viking Press, 1972; Pinnacle Books, 1975).

Pelletier, Kenneth, *Mind As Healer, Mind as Slayer* (New York: Delacorte Press/Delta Books, 1977).

Chapter 6: ALTERNATIVE MEDICINE

This chapter of lists was formed from books of lists. I have experienced personally or have talked with persons who have experienced nearly all of the healing activities in the lists. One of my most persistent impressions is that my lists contain many alternate paths to the same place.

The following books are recommended for the reader who wishes to explore further:

Brodsky, Greg, *From Eden to Aquarius* (New York: Bantam Books, 1974).

Inglis, Brian, *Fringe Medicine* (London: Faber and Faber, 1964).

Kloss, Jethro, *Back to Eden* (Simi Valley, Calif.: Benedict Lust Publications, 1976).

Law, Donald, *A Guide to Alternative Medicine* (New York: Hippocrene Books, 1975).

Loomis, E. G., and Paulson, J. S., *Healing for Everyone: Medicine of the Whole Person* (New York: Hawthorn Books, 1975).

Kiernan, Thomas, *Shrinks, etc.: A Consumer's Guide to Psychotherapies* (New York: Dial Press, 1974; Dell, 1976).

Kruger, Helen, *Other Healers, Other Cures: A Guide to Alternative Medicine* (New York: Bobbs-Merrill, 1974).

Miller, D. M., *Bodymind: The Whole Person Health Book* (Englewood Cliffs, N.J.: Prentice-Hall, 1974); Pinnacle Books, 1975).

Nolen, W. A., *Healing: A Doctor in Search of a Miracle* (New York: Random House, 1975; Fawcett, 1976).

Turner, R. N., *Naturopathic First Aid* (London: Thorsons Publishers, Ltd., 1969).

Wallnofer, H., and von Rottauscher, A., *Chinese Folk Medicine* (New York: New American Library: Mentor, 1974).

Westlake, A. T., *The Pattern of Health: A Search for a Greater Understanding of the Life Force in Health and Disease* (Berkeley: Shambhala Publications, 1973).

Spiritual Community Guide (San Rafael, Calif.: Spiritual Community Publications, 1974).

Chapter 7: HEALING THE BODY

In sheer bulk of literature, nothing exceeds the material on the study of the human body. This most accessible aspect of a human being, the tangible mechanical structure, remains, however, a mysterious subject and a constant source of controversy among researchers. This chapter is intended to demonstrate a variety of different views of body functioning and maintenance, a demonstration that can be continued in the following suggested reading:

Bean, Orson, *Me and the Orgone* (New York: Fawcett Publications, 1971).

Bieler, H. G., *Food Is Your Best Medicine* (New York: Random House: Vintage, 1973).

Chapman, Esther, *How to Use the Twelve Tissue Salts* (New York: Pyramid Publications, 1971).

Coon, Nelson, *Using Plants for Healing* (New York: Hearthside Press, 1963).

222

Coulter, H. L., *Homeopathic Medicine* (Washington, D.C.: American Foundation for Homeopathy, 1972).

Miller, D. E., *Bodymind: The Whole Person Health Book* (Englewood Cliffs, N.J.: Prentice-Hall, 1974; Pinnacle Books, 1975).

Mills, D. L., *Study of Chiropractors, Osteopaths and Naturopaths in Canada* (Ottawa: Queen's Printer, 1966).

Tansley, D. V., *Radionics and the Subtle Anatomy of Man* (Northamptonshire: Health Science Press, 1972).

Vithoulkas, George, *Homeopathy* (New York: Avon Books, 1971).

Chiropractic in California, a report by Stanford Research Institute, South Passadena, Calif. (Los Angeles: The Hayes Foundation, 1960).

Chapter 8: HEALING THE MIND

To some readers a chapter on "mental health" may seem inappropriate, but for most of us to this point seeing a therapist for emotional problems has meant seeing a psychiatrist who is trained as a physician and whose analytic techniques are based on the work of Freud—in other words, an establishment-oriented scientific healer. As defined in the chapter, the variety of mind-healing needs and activities is too wide to be so confined. The following works offer background on some of the many alternatives that are candidates for inclusion in the holistic concept.

Becker, Ernest, *The Denial of Death* (New York: The Free Press, 1973).

Chertok, L., *Hypnosis* (New York: Pergamon Press, 1965).

Ford, Donald H., and Urban, Hugh B., *Systems of Psychotherapy: A Comparative Study* (New York: John Wiley, 1963).

Frank, Jerome, *Persuasion and Healing: A Comparative Study of Psychotherapy* (Baltimore: Johns Hopkins Press, 1973; Schocken Books, 1974).

Inglis, Brian, *Fringe Medicine* (London: Faber and Faber, 1964).

Jones, H. L., et al., *Science and Theory of Health* (Dubuque: W. C. Brown Co., 1966).

Kierman, Thomas, *Shrinks, etc.: A Consumer's Guide to Psychotherapies* (New York: Dial Press, 1974; Dell, 1976).

Kruger, Helen, *Other Healers, Other Cures: A Guide to Alternative Medicine* (New York: Bobbs-Merrill, 1974).

Lowen, Alexander, *Bioenergetics* (New York: Coward, McCann & Geoghegan, 1975; Penguin Books, 1976).

Rawcliff, D. H., *Illusions and Delusions of the Supernatural and the Occult* (New York: Dover Publications, 1959).

Chapter 9: HEALING THE SPIRIT

Among the chapters of this book this is my personal favorite, probably because my spiritual development is now my deepest interest. Yet trying to write analytically and rationally about spirituality turned out to be very difficult, and I chose to emphasize the work of Peter Ford, which has had great influence on my thinking. His *The Healing Trinity* (New York: Harper & Row, 1971) is highly recommended for further reading.

The following books are also recommended for the reader who wishes to explore this subject. They show the wide variety of means by which truly spiritual persons attain, exhibit, and live spiritual lives—no special credentials are necessary.

Cayce, Edgar, *Edgar Cayce on Atlantis* (New York: Warner Books, 1968).

Dooley, Anne, *Every Wall a Door* (New York: E. P. Dutton, 1974).

Edwards, Harry, *The Healing Intelligence* (New York: Taplinger, 1971; Hawthorn Books, 1974).

Hewitt, Cecil R., *Believe What You Like* (London: Andre Deutsch, 1973).

Inglis, Brian, *Fringe Medicine* (London: Faber and Faber, 1964).

Kelsey, Morton, *Healing and Christianity* (New York: Harper & Row, 1976).

Kruger, Helen, *Other Healers, Other Cures: A Guide to Alternative Medicine* (New York: Bobbs-Merrill, 1974).

Loomis, E. G., and Paulson, J. S., *Healing for Everyone: Medicine of the Whole Person* (New York: Hawthorn Books, 1975).

Major, Ralph H., *Faiths That Healed* (New York: Appleton-Century, 1940).

Podmore, Frank, *From Mesmer to Christian Science* (New Hyde Park: University Books, 1963).

Sechrist, Elsie, *Dreams, Your Magic Mirror, with Interpretations of Edgar Cayce* (Chicago: Contemporary Books, 1968; New York: Warner Books, 1974).

Sigerist, Henry E., *Civilization and Disease* (Chicago: University of Chicago Press, 1962).

Chapter 10: SELF-HEALING

The ability to self-heal is both the most basic and the most advanced health process. It seems that self-healing is a skill that has been civilized out of most of us. Some kind of deprogramming is needed to allow our natural skills to re-assert themselves. Any deprogramming requires a significant developmental effort from an individual. Many of the books on the following list are intended to help with that effort.

Back, Linda, *Awake! Aware! Alive!* (New York: Random House, 1973).

Baudouin, Charles, *Suggestion and Autosuggestion* (Norwood, Pa.: Norwood Editions, reprint of 1920 ed.).

Coué, Emile, and Brooks, C. H., *Better and Better Every Day* (New York: Barnes & Noble, 1961).

Rosenberg, Jack L., *Total Orgasm* (New York and Berkeley: Random House/Bookworks, 1973).

Rush, Anne Kent, *Getting Clear* (New York and Berkeley: Random House/Bookworks, 1973).

Samuels, Mike, and Bennett, Hal, *The Well-Body Book* (New York and Berkeley: Random House/Bookworks, 1973).

Samuels, Mike, and Bennett, Hal, *Be Well* (New York and Berkeley: Random House/Bookworks, 1974).

Simmons, Leo (Ed.), *Sun Chief: The Autobiography of a Hopi Indian,* Rev. Ed. (New Haven: Yale University Press, 1963).

Sobel, David, and Hornbacher, Faith, *To Your Health* (New York and Berkeley: Random House/Bookworks, 1973).

Van Dusen, Wilson, *The Natural Depth in Man: A Searcher's Guide for Exploring the Secret Spaces of Our Inner Worlds* (New York: Harper & Row, 1973).

Chapter 11: THE FUTURE

A dream of the future: a place where we can go, present ourselves totally, and heal ourselves totally. It is likely that we will find such a place only in the long-term future beyond the health maintenance organizations and the national health insurance schemes of the short term; and until holistic medicine is institutionalized, people will continue to simulate holistic medicine themselves, thus creating a valuable bank of experience and increasing the pressure for holistic health institutions.

Sources for material cited in this chapter:

Alexander, George, "Tension," *San Francisco Chronicle,* July 14, 1975, p. 15.

Duhl, Leonard, "The Process of Re-Creation," an unpublished paper.

Emerson, H. E., "Prevention Is Better Than Cure," *Journal of the Canadian Medical Association,* Vol. 107, September 9, 1972, pp. 393–394.

Hatch, T. P., "Priorities in Preventive Medicine," *Archives of Environmental Health*, Vol. 29, July 1974, pp. 52–55.

Henderson, C. W., *Awakening: Ways to Psycho-Spiritual Growth* (Englewood Cliffs, N.J.: Prentice-Hall, 1975).

Lowis, Thomas, "An Indian Healer's Preventive Melicine Procedure," *Hospital and Community Psychiatry*, Vol. 25, No. 2, February 1974, pp. 94–95.

Marin, Peter, "The New Narcissism," *Harper's*, Vol. 251, No. 1505, October, 1975.

Morris, S. M., "What We Have Is An Illness System," *Trustee*, July 1970, pp. 18–21.

Nader, Ralph, "Responsibility of Physicians to Society," *Federation Proceedings*, Vol. 31, No. 6, November–December 1972, pp. 1578–1581.

Samuels, Mike, and Bennett, Hal, *The Well-Body Book* (New York and Berkeley: Random House/Bookworks, 1973).

Shindell, Sidney, "Trends in Health Care Delivery," *Preventive Medicine*, Vol. 1, 1972, pp. 547–553.

Wise, Harold, "The Family Center," an unpublished proposal.

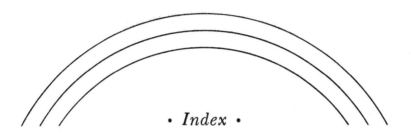

Index

Rankian, 111–112
rational, 112
Reichian, 101, 105, 112, 173
sex, 101–102
sleep, 102
vitamin, 103, 182
see also Analysis, Healing,
    Scientific medicine
Tillich, Paul, 164
To a Dancing God (Keen), 178
Touching, 21, 62, 115–116, 130,
    134
Traditional medicine: *see*
    Scientific medicine
Trauma of Birth, The (Rank),
    111–112
Transactional analysis, 113, 154
Transcendental Meditation,
    149, 151
Tranquilizers, 40, 197
Trousseau, Armand, 87
Travis, John, 213
Tuberculosis, 6, 50, 127, 183, 184
Twitchell, Paul, 116

Ulcer, 63, 67, 81, 109, 133, 166
Ulcer diet, 90
Unani medicine, 103

Vaccination: *see* Immunization
Vascular disease, 4
Vegetarianism, 16–17, 34, 103,
    190
Ventilation, 38
Vietnam War, 10
Vitamin therapy, 103, 182
Voodoo, 32, 39–41, 120

Waiting room, 20
Well Body Book, The (Samuels
    and Bennett), 179, 193–194
Wellness Resource Center (Mill
    Valley, Calif.), 213
Wesley, John, 40
Wholistic Health Center
    (Hinsdale, Ill.), 213
Wise, Harold, 208–209, 212
Witch doctors, 2, 24–25, 51, 53

X ray, 66

Yoga, 76, 82, 99, 101, 103, 113–
    114, 116, 119, 144, 153, 168,
    173, 210

Zen, 120
Zen macrobiotics, 103